Questions and Answers in Magnetic Resonance Imaging

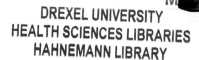
Questions and Answers in

MAGNETIC RESONANCE IMAGING

ALLEN D. ELSTER, M.D.

Professor of Radiology
Co-Director of MR Imaging
Bowman Gray School of Medicine
Wake Forest University
Winston-Salem, North Carolina

With 111 illustrations

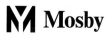 **Mosby**

St. Louis   Baltimore   Boston   Chicago   London   Madrid   Philadelphia   Sydney   Toronto

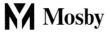
Mosby

Dedicated to Publishing Excellence

Editor: Robert J. Farrell
Editorial Assistant: Andrea M. Whitson
Project Manager: Peggy Fagen
Production Editor: Roger McWilliams
Designer: Elizabeth Rohne Rudder

**WN
185
E49q
1994**

Printed in the United States of America
Composition by Graphic World
Printing/binding by Maple-Vail Book Manufacturing Group

Mosby–Year Book, Inc.
11830 Westline Industrial Drive
St. Louis, Missouri 63146

International Standard Book Number 0-8016-7767-X

93 94 95 96 97 GW/MY 9 8 7 6 5 4 3 2 1

To Allen, Elizabeth, Martha, and Patricia—

Keep asking those questions.

Preface

Over the last 6 years, I have had the pleasure of teaching the physical principles of magnetic resonance (MR) imaging to hundreds of technologists, residents, fellows, and visiting physicians who have participated in educational programs sponsored by the Bowman Gray School of Medicine. Like experienced teachers in other disciplines, I came to realize that each group of students struggled with many of the same conceptual problems year after year. Because I was being asked many of the same questions over and over again, I found myself repeatedly giving the same lectures and explanations to each group of new students. Eventually I developed a series of handouts and drawings that I would distribute and discuss when certain common questions arose. As these handouts became more numerous and sophisticated, they began to form the basis for the book you are now reading, *Questions and Answers in Magnetic Resonance Imaging*.

At least three quarters of the questions in this book were at one time directly posed to me by students, being retained in their original (and sometimes awkward) form as best I can remember them. The remaining 25% of questions are of my own construction; these are questions that I often ask students in order to reinforce their basic understanding of MR physics and to force them to reflect more critically on certain key concepts.

Since the mid 1980s, when I published the first whole-body MR atlas* and first textbook devoted exclusively to cranial MR imaging,† numerous other MR books and teaching aids have become available. *Questions and*

---

*Elster AD: Magnetic resonance imaging. A reference guide and atlas, Philadelphia, 1986, Lippincott.
†Elster AD: Cranial magnetic resonance imaging, New York, 1987, Churchill Livingstone.

Answers in Magnetic Resonance Imaging is intended to supplement, not replace, these larger texts. Each answer is purposefully limited to a few paragraphs, and only a pertinent reference or two from the literature are cited. For the most part, I have included material that is highly practical and immediately applicable to clinical MR imaging. Occasionally, however, I will delve into topics that are principally of historical interest or represent a future direction for MR. Hopefully, these excursions into the past and future will add some color and spirit to MR physics that I try to convey to students in my live lectures.

The book is primarily intended for readers with some clinical knowledge of MR imaging who desire to know more about the physical basis of what they see. While MR specialists may already know the answers to many of these questions, I daresay even they will benefit from a few points scattered throughout this text. Just to be sure, I have included a few tough questions especially for them!

Good luck to all.

Allen D. Elster

Contents

1 **Basic Principles of Electricity and Magnetism,** *1*

2 **Introduction to Nuclear Magnetic Resonance,** *22*

3 **Scanner Hardware,** *62*

4 **Creating an MR Image,** *79*

5 **Gradient Echo Imaging,** *112*

6 **MR Artifacts,** *134*

7 **Flow Phenomena and MR Angiography,** *162*

8 **MR Contrast Agents,** *189*

9 **Advanced MR Imaging Techniques,** *208*

10 **Safety and Biological Effects,** *240*

Appendix, *261*

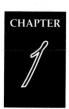

Basic Principles of Electricity and Magnetism

To understand the more complex aspects of magnetic resonance (MR) physics, it is first necessary to review some basic principles of electricity and magnetism you may have forgotten (or never learned) in high school or college. Although most of the individual equations presented in this chapter are *not* important, the basic concepts and definitions *are*.

Part of the confusion with electromagnetic terminology in many MR textbooks arises from two different systems of measurement often being intermixed: the older *centimeter-gram-second (CGS)*, or *gaussian, system* and the more modern *meter-kilogram-second-ampere (MKSA) system*, also called the *Système International d'Unités (SI)*. These two systems differ not only in their nomenclature and units of measurement but also in their definitions of several fundamental electromagnetic quantities. For interested and advanced students, some of these subtle distinctions are addressed in Q 1.07.

Q 1.01	The field strength of our MR scanner is said to be 1.5 tesla. How large is a tesla, and what exactly does this mean?

The strength of a magnetic field is operationally defined in terms of the deflecting force the field exerts on a current or electrical charge moving through it. With reference to Fig. 1-1, consider a hypothetical wire stretched across the bore of an MR scanner whose magnetic field lines

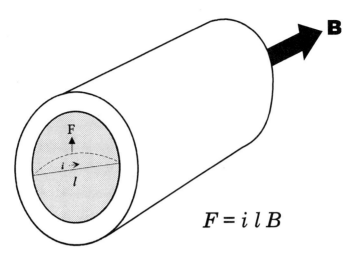

$$F = i\,l\,B$$

Fig. 1-1. Definition of magnetic strength *(B)*. A hypothetical wire of length *l* carrying a current *i* perpendicular to *B* experiences a force *F* given by the equation $F = i\,l\,B$.

are directed along the bore. When a current is passed through this wire, a magnetically generated force deflects the wire upward. The magnitude of this force *(F)* is proportional to the current *(i)*, the length of the wire *(l)*, and the strength of the magnetic field *(B)*. If the wire is exactly perpendicular to the lines of the magnetic field, the force is maximal and is given by

$$F = i\,l\,B$$

We see from this equation that *B* should be expressed in units of force ÷ (current × distance). The SI units for *B* are therefore newtons per ampere-meter, or *tesla (T)*. In other words, an ideal wire carrying a current of 1 ampere perpendicular to a magnetic field of 1 T experiences a deflecting force of 1 newton along each meter of its length.

In the older CGS system, *B* is measured in *gauss (G)*. For conversion, 1 T equals 10,000 G. Because the tesla is a relatively large unit, it is most suitably used to define the strength of the *main* magnetic field of an MR scanner. *Subsystems* (such as gradient coils) within the MR imager generate much smaller fields more conveniently measured in gauss.

The reader should realize that we have defined only the *magnitude (B)* of the field at a given point. If the field is perfectly uniform, *B* is the same at all points within the field. In general, however, the structure of the magnetic field is more complex, and *B* may have different values and directions of action at different points in space. A magnetic field is therefore formally defined to be an array of vectors (denoted by the boldfaced letter **B**) whose size and direction at each point in space define how the field will act on a charge moving at that location.

Reference

Weidner RT, Sells RL. Elementary classical physics, 2nd ed. Boston: Allyn and Bacon, 1973, pp 572-598. (A similar discussion can be found in most college-level physics texts.)

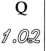

Q **I still don't have a clear idea of how large a 1.5-tesla magnetic field really is. How much stronger is it than a refrigerator magnet or the big magnet in a junkyard that picks up cars?**

Although a 1.5 T scanner is considered "high field" compared with other *imaging* devices, this field strength is actually "midrange" when judged against other experimental and commercial applications of magnets. High-resolution nuclear magnetic resonance (NMR) spectrometers used in chemistry laboratories typically possess much higher fields than clinical MR imagers, usually in the 2 T to 11 T range; a few research sites have specially constructed NMR spectrometers operating at up to 14 T. The large electromagnets that pick up junk cars and scrap metal have fields of 1.5 T to 2.0 T, but they are extremely inhomogeneous (nonuniform). By comparison, a household refrigerator magnet generates a field of less than 10 millitesla (mT) (100 G). The Earth's magnetic field is even smaller, varying from about 30 microtesla (μT) (0.3 G) at the equator to about 70 μT (0.7 G) at the poles.

Q **What is the orientation of the main magnetic field within an MR scanner?**

Commercially available MR scanners have either horizontally or vertically oriented main magnetic fields (Fig. 1-2). All superconducting and most resistive scanners are of solenoidal design, and their main magnetic fields are directed along the bore of the magnet. In some lower-field permanent and resistive scanners, however, the magnetic fields are oriented vertically.

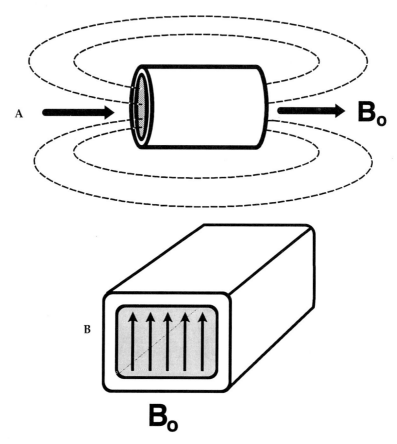

Fig. 1-2. **A,** Most resistive and superconducting MR imagers have their main magnetic fields **(B₀)** directed along the scanner bores. **B,** A few permanent magnet scanners have a vertical orientation of their fields.

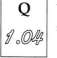

Q	Does it matter which end of an MR scanner is the north or south pole?
1.04	

For a single scanner the answer is "no"; the actual field direction (from front to back or back to front) is irrelevant. When two or more scanners are sited near each other, however, the answer is "yes," and some consideration should be given to polarity of each magnet. In general, magnetic fringe fields and interactions are minimized by configuring the magnets so that the unlike poles face each other.

Q

What is meant by a magnetic field gradient?

1.05

When the strength or direction of a magnetic field differs between two points in space, a *magnetic field gradient* is said to exist. This gradient is defined as the rate at which magnetic field strength changes with position. For example, if a magnetic field increases in magnitude by 0.001 T over a distance of 1 meter (m), the magnetic field gradient would be 0.001 T/m or 1 mT/m in that direction.

By definition, an ideal, perfectly homogeneous magnetic field contains no gradients. In any real field, however, inhomogeneities (and thus magnetic field gradients) must occur. These magnetic gradients may result from (1) intrinsic imperfections in the field itself, known as *static field inhomogeneities*, (2) the presence of matter within the field, whose charged particles interact with the field to create *susceptibility gradients*, or (3) the purposeful activation of specialized gradient coils that create predictable distortions of the main magnetic field and allow spatial encoding of the MR signal. Static field inhomogeneities are discussed in Chapter 2 and susceptibility effects in Q 1.06 to Q 1.10. In this section I address the purposeful type of magnetic field gradients used for imaging.

Imaging gradients are produced by special electrical windings, known as *gradient coils*, that are housed within the body of the MR imager. When energized with electricity, these coils create additional small magnetic fields that distort the main magnetic field as a function of position within the scanner. Typically, there are three sets of such coils (x-, y-, and z-) corresponding to the cardinal directions within the scanner. By convention, the z-axis is usually taken to coincide with the direction of the main magnetic field ($\mathbf{B_o}$), which may be either parallel or perpendicular to the gantry, depending on scanner design (see Q 1.03 and Fig. 1-2).

When a certain gradient is turned on, it creates a predictable distortion of the magnitude, *but not the direction*, of $\mathbf{B_o}$ along that axis. In other words, the magnetic field lines always retain their original orientations (parallel to the z-axis) even when the x-gradient or y-gradient coils are energized. It is thus only the magnitude of $\mathbf{B_o}$ in the z-direction that varies spatially according to position along the x- or y-axis. (In mathematical terms, the x-, y-, and z-gradients are altering $\partial B_z/\partial x$, $\partial B_z/\partial y$, and $\partial B_z/\partial z$, respectively.) These concepts are illustrated graphically in Fig. 1-3.

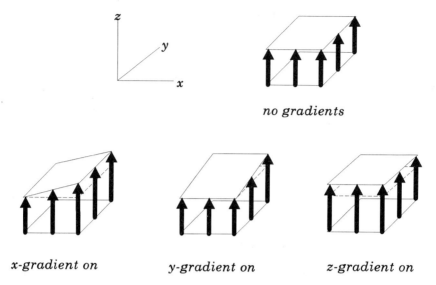

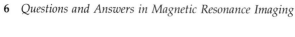

Fig. 1-3. Magnetic field gradients along each of the cardinal scanner directions (x, y, and z).

Q 1.06	In some textbooks I've seen two different designations for the magnetic field, B and H. What's the difference between them?

This relatively advanced question is sometimes raised by MR fellows who have encountered these two magnetic field designations in their readings. Novice students of MR should feel free to skip the moderately technical answer to this question and proceed directly to Q 1.07. For students who are interested, the difference between **B** and **H** fields is discussed in the following paragraphs, with the hope that this explanation clarifies some confusing concepts about SI and CGS units as well.

The magnetic field (**B**) defined in Q 1.01 is also known as the *magnetic induction field*, *magnetic induction*, or *magnetic flux density*. However, another type of magnetic field, denoted by **H**, is called the *magnetic field intensity*. **H** and **B** have different units and a different physical significance. **H** may be thought of as an externally applied *"magnetizing force,"* whereas **B** represents the actual magnetic field *induced* within a region of space. It is necessary to distinguish between **H** and **B** because the electromagnetic field at a given point in space depends not only on the distribution of electrical currents giving rise to that field (reflected in **H**) but also on the type of matter occupying the region (reflected in **B**).

When no matter is present (i.e., in a vacuum), **B** and **H** are essentially equivalent, except for a factor μ_o to adjust units of measurement. Thus, we can write: $\mathbf{B_{vac}} = \mu_o\mathbf{H}$. The factor μ_o is called the *permeability of free space* and has the value $4\pi \times 10^{-7}$ newtons/ampere^2 in SI units. Since **B** is measured in tesla (newtons per ampere-meter), the SI units for **H** must therefore be amperes per meter. In the CGS system, however, μ_o is dimensionless and is assigned the value 1. In the CGS system, therefore, both **B** and **H** are measured in the same units (gauss), although they continue to have a different physical significance. (To complicate matters even more, sometimes the CGS unit for **H** has been called the oersted [Oe]; however, since 1 Oe = 1 G, there seems to be little point in perpetuating this even older nomenclature.)

Whenever matter is present within a given region of space, the induced field (**B**) is generally not equal to the applied field (**H**). When **H** encounters matter, various electromagnetic interactions occur that can be thought of as tending to "concentrate" or "disperse" the magnetic lines of force. This phenomenon results primarily from the action of unpaired orbital and delocalized electrons, which set up circulating currents and secondarily induce an internal *magnetization* (**M**$_i$) within the matter that serves either to augment or to oppose the applied field (**H**).

In matter, therefore, the relationship between **B** and **H** is quite complex but can be approximated by the relationship

$$\mathbf{B} = \mu_o\,\mu\,\mathbf{H}$$

where μ is a dimensionless factor known as the *relative magnetic permeability* of the material. When $\mu > 1$ the magnetic field can be thought of as "concentrated" relative to that in a vacuum. When $\mu < 1$ the field can be considered relatively "thinned" or "dispersed" within the matter. Substances with $\mu > 1$ are called *paramagnetic*; those with $\mu < 1$ are called *diamagnetic*. These concepts are discussed in greater detail in Q 1.07.

The relative permeability of a material, μ, is closely related to another dimensionless property known as *magnetic susceptibility*. The defining formulae and symbols used in the SI system differ slightly from those used in the CGS system, as follows:

$$\mu = 1 + \kappa \text{ (SI)} \quad \text{and} \quad \mu = 1 + 4\pi\chi \text{ (CGS)}$$

where κ in the SI system and χ in the CGS system are termed *volume magnetic susceptibilities*. For purposes of conversion between the SI and CGS systems, $\kappa = 4\pi\chi$. Under this alternative formulation, paramagnetic substances are said to have positive susceptibilities, and diamagnetic substances have negative susceptibilities.

We may further define the induced *magnetization* (**M**$_i$) per unit volume of a substance as

$$\mathbf{M_i} = \kappa\,\mathbf{H}\ \text{(SI) and } \mathbf{M_i} = \chi\,\mathbf{H}\ \text{(CGS)}$$

For paramagnetic substances ($\kappa, \chi > 0$), $\mathbf{M_i}$ points in the same direction as $\mathbf{H}$, and the "effective field" is thus augmented. For diamagnetic substances ($\kappa, \chi > 0$), $\mathbf{M_i}$ and $\mathbf{H}$ point in opposite directions, and the effective field is thus diminished.

Some chemistry textbooks and MR articles do not report κ and χ in their volumetric (dimensionless) forms but rather as *mass susceptibilities* (κ_m or χ_m) or *molar susceptibilities* (κ_M or χ_M), which *do* have dimensions (cubic centimeters per gram and cubic centimeters per mole, respectively). Additionally, $\mathbf{M_i}$ is sometimes defined *per unit mass or mole* and therefore has different dimensions from those used here. One need not memorize a dozen different equations and definitions; the important point is that these quantities and concepts are expressed in different ways in different textbooks and articles. I will continue to use the more widely accepted dimensionless forms of κ and χ throughout this book and urge other authors to do the same.

The relationships among $\mathbf{B}$, $\mathbf{M_i}$, and $\mathbf{H}$ in the SI and CGS systems can now be formally expressed by combining the previous equations:

$$\mathbf{B} = \mu_o\,\mu\,\mathbf{H} = \mu_o\,(1 + \kappa)\,\mathbf{H} = \mu_o\,(\mathbf{H} + \kappa\mathbf{H}) = \mu_o\,(\mathbf{H} + \mathbf{M_i})\ \text{(SI)}$$

$$\mathbf{B} = \mu_o\,\mu\,\mathbf{H} = 1 \cdot (1 + 4\pi\chi)\,\mathbf{H} = \mathbf{H} + 4\pi\chi\mathbf{H} = \mathbf{H} + 4\pi\mathbf{M_i}\ \text{(CGS)}$$

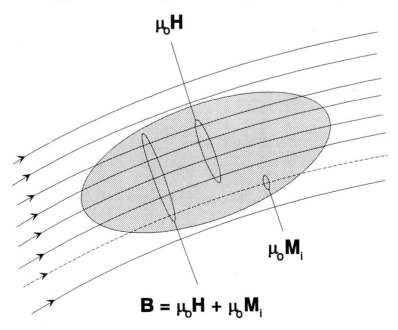

Fig. 1-4. Relationship between **B** and **H** fields in matter (*gray oval*). See Q 1.06 for details.

| TABLE | 1-1. Fundamental Units of Electromagnetism |

Property	Symbol	SI Units	CGS Units
Magnetic induction field (flux density)	B	Tesla	Gauss
Magnetic field intensity	H	Ampere per meter	Gauss (oersted)
Magnetization	M_i	Ampere per meter	Gauss
Permeability of free space	μ_o	$4\pi \times 10^{-7}$ newtons/ampere^2	1 (dimensionless)
Relative magnetic permeability	μ	Dimensionless	Dimensionless
Volume magnetic susceptibility	κ, X	Dimensionless	Dimensionless

These relationships among **B**, **M$_i$**, and **H** are illustrated graphically in Fig. 1-4. The names and units of several fundamental magnetic properties in the SI and CGS systems are summarized in Table 1-1.

Reference

Lentner C (ed). Geigy scientific tables, 8th ed. Vol 1. Units of measurement, body fluids, composition of the body, nutrition. Summit, NJ: Ciba-Geigy, 1981, pp 9-28.

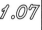
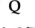

Q **What is magnetic susceptibility?**

Magnetic susceptibility is a measure of the extent to which a substance becomes magnetized when it is placed in an external magnetic field. Magnetic susceptibility is therefore sometimes referred to as *magnetizability*.

Whenever matter is placed in a magnetic field, electromagnetic interactions take place between the matter and the field. These interactions "concentrate" or "disperse" the lines of the magnetic field (Fig. 1-5). This phenomenon results principally from the action within the matter of orbital and delocalized electrons, which set up circulating currents in response to the externally applied field. These circulating currents, in turn, induce within the matter an internal magnetization (**M$_i$**) that either augments or opposes the external field. When the direction of **M$_i$** is the same as that of the external field, effective field within the object is enhanced. This magnetic field enhancement phenomenon is known as *paramagnetism*.

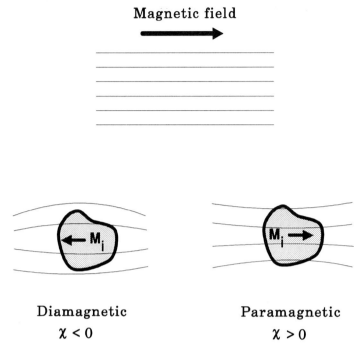

Fig. 1-5. Magnetic susceptibility. Diamagnetic substances have negative susceptibilities ($\chi < 0$) and act to "disperse" the lines of the externally applied field. Paramagnetic substances have positive susceptibilities ($\chi > 0$) and tend to "concentrate" the lines of the field, thus increasing its local value.

When the direction of $\mathbf{M_i}$ is opposite to that of the external field, the effective field within the object is reduced, and the effect is known as *diamagnetism*.

Magnetic susceptibility is defined as the magnitude of $\mathbf{M_i}$ divided by the strength of the external field. Susceptibility is typically denoted by the Greek symbol χ (or κ). For most biological materials, χ is a small number (on the order of 10^{-4} to 10^{-6}), so the difference between the magnetic field in a vacuum and that in tissue is relatively slight. However, some materials (such as iron) possess extremely large values for χ (~10,000). The induced field within iron can therefore be substantially greater than in a vacuum; therefore, iron is suitable for use in such applications as transformers and electromagnets. Depending on their exact magnetic properties, materials with large positive susceptibilities may be termed *superparamagnetic* or *ferromagnetic*. These concepts are summarized in Table 1-2 and are discussed in greater detail in Q 1.08 and Q 1.09.

| | **TABLE** | **1-2. Magnetic Properties of Matter** | |

Magnetic Property	Direction of Magnetization Relative to External Field	Relative Magnetic Susceptibility	Typical Materials
Diamagnetism	Opposite	−1	Water, most organic molecules, salts of nonmetals, inert gases
Paramagnetism	Same	+10	Ions, simple salts and chelates of metals (Cr, Fe, Mn, Co, Cu, Gd, Dy), molecular O_2, organic free radicals
Superparamagnetism	Same	+5000	Small Fe_3SO_4 particles
Ferromagnetism	Same	+25,000	Larger Fe_3SO_4 particles, multi-domain metals and alloys (Fe, Ni, Co)

Reference

Saini S, Frankel RB, Stark DD, Ferrucci JT Jr. Magnetism: a primer and review. AJR 150:735, 1988. (Although this is a good general reference for concepts pertaining to magnetic susceptibility, the authors include a confusing mix of CGS and SI units in their discussion, with resulting inconsistencies in some of their definitions and equations.)

Q 1.08

Please explain more about the differences between diamagnetism and paramagnetism.

These two terms, introduced in Q 1.07, are used to classify different materials on the basis of their intrinsic magnetic susceptibilities. These magnetic susceptibility properties, in turn, are determined principally by the number of delocalized and unpaired orbital electrons within the materials (Table 1-2).

The overwhelming majority of organic molecules and simple, nonmetallic compounds are *diamagnetic*. In these materials the induced magnetization opposes the direction of the main magnetic field. Water and most biological tissues are diamagnetic, with susceptibility constants on the order of -1.0×10^{-6}. This weak diamagnetism is primarily caused by the orbital momentum of paired electrons, although spin-orbital coupling to electron spins makes a minor contribution.

Some atoms and many charged molecules possess unpaired electrons in their outer shells. The magnetic moments associated with these electrons tend to align with and thus augment the externally applied field. These ions and molecules have positive values of χ and are termed *paramagnetic*. The rare-earth elements gadolinium (Gd) and dysprosium (Dy) and their complexes are among the strongest paramagnetic substances known because they possess many unpaired electrons in their 4f shells. For ions with half-filled shells whose magnetism comes purely from spin angular momentum (like Gd^{+3} and Mn^{+2}), the degree of expected paramagnetism is proportional to $N(N + 2)$, where N = the number of unpaired electrons.

Some atoms (such as ^1H, ^{31}P, and ^{23}Na) demonstrate paramagnetism only in the immediate vicinity of their nuclei; this is termed *nuclear paramagnetism* and is the basis for the NMR phenomenon. Nuclear paramagnetic effects, however, are generally several thousand times weaker than the paramagnetism or diamagnetism associated with electrons. The overall susceptibility of a substance, therefore, is dominated by electronic rather than nuclear effects.

This concept bears restating: *the bulk magnetic properties of a substance principally result from electrons, whereas the NMR phenomenon involves nuclei (protons and neutrons)*. Thus the individual hydrogen protons in a water molecule demonstrate *nuclear paramagnetism*, meaning their *nuclear* magnetic moments tend to align with the field. As a bulk substance, however, water is *diamagnetic*, and its total induced magnetization points *opposite* to the direction of the applied field.

Reference

Weidner RT, Sells RL. Elementary classical physics, 2nd ed. Boston: Allyn and Bacon, 1973, pp 655-667. (A similar discussion can be found in most college-level physics texts.)

Q	What distinguishes superparamagnetism from paramagnetism? How does each of these differ from ferromagnetism?
1.09	

Electronic effects are even more dominant in the solid or crystalline forms of certain metals, such as iron, nickel, and cobalt. These materials have

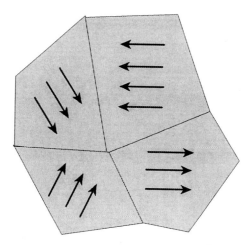

Fig. 1-6. A ferromagnetic substance consists of several magnetic domains, in which all electron spins become locked together because of exchange coupling.

extremely large positive susceptibilities and are termed *ferromagnetic.* Whereas paramagnetism and diamagnetism are properties of individual atoms or molecules, ferromagnetism is a property of a group of atoms or molecules in a solid crystal or lattice. All ferromagnetic substances have unpaired electron spins that are strongly entwined by a quantum mechanical force, *exchange coupling,* for which there is no classical analog. As a consequence of exchange coupling, large groups of atoms in a ferromagnetic substance form magnetic *domains,* in which all electron spins become locked together in alignment (Fig. 1-6).

The formation of magnetic domains accounts for the extremely large values of χ observed in ferromagnetic materials; it also gives them a "magnetic memory," or *remanence,* in which the actual value of χ depends on the past magnetization history of the material. Iron, for example, can retain appreciable residual magnetization even after the external magnetic field has been removed. This magnetic memory is one reason iron and iron alloys are frequently chosen for making permanent magnets.

Superparamagnetism is more closely related to ferromagnetism than to paramagnetism. Superparamagnetism occurs principally in small, single-domain magnetic particles. For example, when a ferromagnetic, multidomain sample of Fe_3O_4 is reduced in size to less than about 350 angstroms (Å), a single-domain magnetic particle eventually will be formed. When placed in an external magnetic field, this particle develops a strong internal magnetization from exchange coupling of electrons within the domain and thus becomes *super*paramagnetic. Because only a single domain is

TABLE 1-3. Comparison of Superparamagnetism and Ferromagnetism		
	Superparamagnetism	Ferromagnetism
Structure	Single-domain particle	Multiple domains
Magnetic memory	No	Yes
Degree of induced magnetism	Moderate	Very high

involved, the susceptibility of a superparamagnetic substance is not nearly as great as that of a ferromagnetic substance. Additionally, since each domain is in a separate particle, there can be no interactions or ordering of domains within a sample. Unlike ferromagnetic materials, therefore, superparamagnetic substances do not retain any net magnetization once the external field has been removed. In other words, they have no magnetic memory. Table 1-3 compares superparamagnetism and ferromagnetism.

Q 1.10   What is a magnetic susceptibility gradient?

Biological tissues often contain materials with different intrinsic susceptibilities that are anatomically juxtaposed. For example, the susceptibilities of air, bone, and cerebrospinal fluid (CSF) differ greatly. At sharp interfaces, for example, between the brain and sphenoid sinus or between CSF and vertebral bodies, rapid local variations in χ (and thus **B**) occur. These local variations in the magnetic field are termed *susceptibility gradients* and are responsible for both artifacts and signal losses during clinical MR imaging (see Q 6.05).

Tissue susceptibility gradients may also exist when either endogenous or exogenous paramagnetic materials accumulate focally within tissues. Endogenously occurring paramagnetic substances include certain blood degradation products (deoxyhemoglobin, methemoglobin, hemosiderin, ferritin) and the pigment melanin. Exogenously administered paramagnetic substances include gadolinium, manganese, and iron compounds used as MR contrast agents. These substances are capable of inducing large susceptibility gradients between different tissue compartments.

Reference

Elster AD. Sellar susceptibility artifacts: theory and implications. AJNR 14:129, 1993.

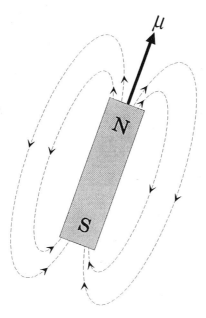

Fig. 1-7. In the magnetic dipole (μ) concept, local magnetic fields from subatomic particles, ions, and small molecules are considered to emanate from a tiny bar magnet or current loop at the center of the particle.

Q	**What is a magnetic dipole?**
1.11	

A magnetic dipole is a *concept* used in physics to model the emanation of local magnetic fields from individual molecular, atomic, and subatomic sources (e.g., ions, protons, electrons). For convenience, the magnetic dipole can be visualized as a tiny bar magnet with north and south poles (Fig. 1-7). The vector representation of this "point-source" magnetic field is typically denoted by **μ** and is called the magnetic dipole *moment*.

Because of its much greater ratio of charge to mass, the electron possesses a magnetic moment approximately 1000 times larger than that of a proton. This is the principal reason that electronic effects are so much more important than nuclear ones in explaining the bulk magnetic properties of matter.

The reader should note that the concept of the magnetic dipole is not restricted to the modeling of individual subatomic particles and can be applied to whole nuclei, atoms, and even molecules. A bar magnet and a compass needle might even be considered giant dipoles. The term *dipole-dipole interaction* generally refers to the interaction between two such particles (e.g., between two protons or between a proton and an electron) through their associated dipolar magnetic fields.

> **Q 1.12** | **All the books I read about NMR show protons precessing like little tops or gyroscopes within the magnetic field. I don't really understand why this type of motion should occur. Can you explain?**

Perhaps the action of the proton can be best understood through an analogy with the motion of a compass needle within a magnetic field (Fig. 1-8). We all know that a compass needle naturally seeks to lie parallel to the lines of an external magnetic field (B_o). Furthermore, if the needle is initially placed obliquely within the field, it experiences a torque, or twisting force, that seeks to bring it into alignment. Let us now analyze the motion of this needle under a variety of conditions.

In the first case, let us assume that the needle is initially oriented at some oblique angle to the magnetic field, is constrained to move within a single plane, and has a frictionless pivot point (Fig. 1-8, *A*). Because it is initially oblique, the needle experiences a magnetic torque and thus begins to move. The needle accelerates, actually overshoots its goal of perfect alignment with B_o, and swings to the other side, where it eventually decelerates as a result of torque in the opposite direction. The needle then reverses its course and again swings back, seeking to align with B_o, but again overshoots its mark. In a frictionless system, therefore, the compass needle never aligns with B_o, but instead oscillates indefinitely around B_o with a characteristic frequency, ω_o.

The frequency of oscillation of the compass needle is directly proportional to the strength (B_o) of the magnetic field. If the compass is brought closer to the pole of the magnet, it experiences a stronger field and oscillates faster (Fig. 1-8, *B*). The rate of oscillation also depends on several intrinsic properties of the compass needle (e.g., its mass and shape), which can be combined into a proportionality constant (γ) called the *gyromagnetic ratio*. For this simple compass model, we find that

$$\omega_o = \gamma\, B_o$$

This relationship is known as the Larmor equation and is also applicable to NMR, Zeeman splitting, and a variety of other physical phenomena.

In the next case, let us now relax the restriction that the compass can move in only one plane and give it a three-dimensional (3D) pivot point,

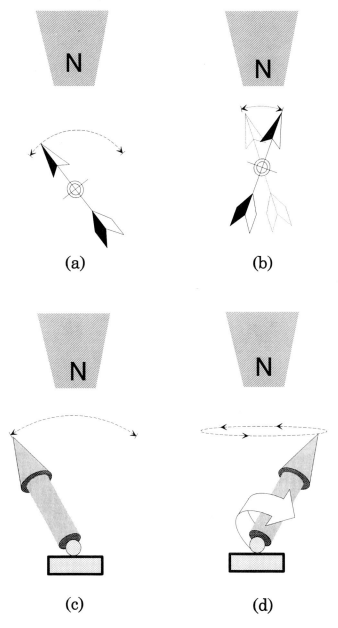

Fig. 1-8. **A,** An ideal compass needle, constrained to frictionless pivoting in a single plane, oscillates indefinitely but never aligns with the north pole *(N).* **B,** If the magnetic pole is brought closer (i.e., the local field is made stronger), the compass needle oscillates more rapidly. **C,** With full three-dimentional pivoting, the compass needle still experiences a planar oscillation when displaced. **D,** Only when given angular momentum (by spinning it around its own axis) will the compass needle undergo a gyroscopic precession around the direction of the external field.

as shown in Fig. 1-8, C. Will the motion of the needle now be a gyroscopic precession? It may be surprising to learn that the answer is still "no." Even with full 3D pivoting, the compass still oscillates only in a single plane when it is displaced.

How then do we get it to precess? We do this by imparting to the compass needle a mechanical property (angular momentum), produced by spinning it similar to a top along its own axis (Fig. 1-8, D). This is directly analogous to the model of the proton found in many books as a "spinning magnet." When our compass needle spins around its own axis, its interaction with the external field is no longer a simple planar oscillation. Although magnetic forces attempt to align the compass with B_o as before, angular momentum considerations dictate that the net effect is a torque, or twisting force, directed perpendicularly to both the needle and B_o. This tangential force causes the compass needle to move in a gyroscopic precession in a cone around the direction of B_o, again with characteristic frequency $\omega_o = \gamma\, B_o$.

This fundamental point needs restating: *precession in a magnetic field requires the coupling and interaction of two different physical properties of the system, electromagnetic and mechanical.*

Q *1.13*	**But a real compass doesn't oscillate indefinitely.**

You are absolutely right. In any real compass, friction is always present at the pivot point. After displacing the needle from its equilibrium alignment, the oscillations we have described will occur, but they die out rapidly. In the 3D case, we would see an early precession, but with time the needle would gradually spiral inward and would eventually align with B_o. This loss of energy through friction is analogous to T1 relaxation in NMR, which is discussed more completely in Chapter 2.

Q *1.14*	**Where does the energy come from to keep the precession going?**

Surprisingly, no energy is required to keep the precession going. The reason for this is not immediately obvious but can be understood by considering how the potential energy of the compass needle varies according to its angle of orientation in the field.

Let us refer again to the model presented in Q 1.12, in which a compass needle (representing the magnetic dipole **μ**) is immersed within an external magnetic field (**B_o**). As previously discussed, the natural tendency of this system is for the compass needle to rest in a direction parallel to B_o. In other words, the total system energy naturally seeks its lowest state, which occurs when the needle is parallel to B_o. To move the needle so that it points away from this natural orientation, one must do work on the needle (by pushing it with a finger). Because any other needle position can be obtained only by adding work/energy to the system (e.g., by pushing on the needle), the potential energies are higher in these orientations than in a state of rest. The maximum system energy occurs when the compass points in a direction exactly opposite to its natural alignment (i.e., μ is antiparallel to B_o).

From this analogy with a compass, we can now understand better some of the energy relationships between magnetic dipoles and magnetic fields. First, system energy is *minimized* when μ is parallel to B_o and *maximized* when μ is antiparallel to B_o. When μ is obliquely oriented to B_o the energy level has some intermediate value that depends on the angle between μ and B_o. Second, we see that energy must be added (or removed) from the system to change the orientation of μ relative to B_o. Third, if the angle between μ and B_o remains constant (as it does during a simple precession), the system energy remains constant. Thus no energy is required to maintain a simple magnetic precession.

| Q 1.15 | **Why did you use the symbol ω_o for precessional frequency?** |

The symbol ω_o represents the *angular frequency* of precession and has units of radians per second. Most readers are more familiar with the concept of *cyclic frequency*, which is denoted by the symbol f_o and measured in cycles per second, or hertz (Hz). Since 2π radians $= 360°$ $= 1$ cycle (revolution), angular and cyclic frequencies can be easily converted by the equation

$$\omega_o = 2 \pi f_o$$

| Q 1.16 | **What is the difference between phase and frequency?** |

Any periodically oscillating wave or signal (like a sine wave) has three fundamental properties: amplitude, frequency, and phase. These properties are explicitly apparent in the mathematical formulation for a sine wave:

$$S(t) = A \, sin(\omega_o t + \phi)$$

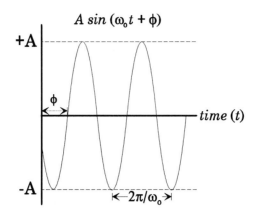

Fig. 1-9. A sine wave is defined mathematically by its amplitude *(A)*, angular frequency (ω_o), and phase (ϕ).

where $S(t)$ is the signal as a function of time, A is the amplitude, ω_o is the angular frequency, and ϕ is the instantaneous phase. By adjusting these factors, the appearance of the sine wave can be varied (Fig. 1-9). Instantaneous phase (ϕ) represents an angular shift between two sine waves and is measured in radians (or degrees). A sine wave and a cosine wave are 90° ($\pi/2$ radians) out of phase with each other.

After a period of time, Δt, two sine waves initially synchronized in phase but differing in frequency by $\Delta\omega$ radians per second will develop a differential total phase shift $(\Delta\Phi)$ given by:

$$\Delta\Phi = \Delta\omega \cdot \Delta t$$

In more general terms expressed by calculus:

$$\Phi = \int \omega \, dt$$

The total accumulated phase (Φ) can be thought of as the area under a frequency-versus-time curve. This fact is useful when we discuss phase changes resulting from flow in Chapter 7.

In MR imaging the signals we record are in the form of "sine" waves that vary in frequency and phase according to their site of emanation within the subject. Furthermore, we do not measure the signal from individual protons but instead record a summation of many such signals originating from protons within an entire volume of interest.

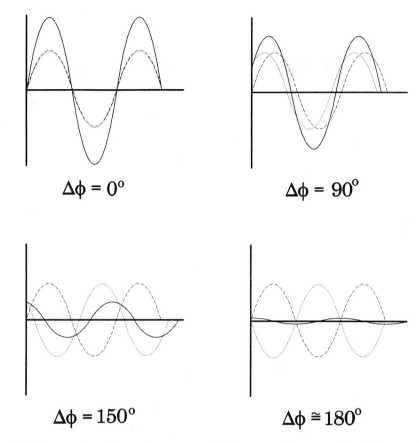

$$\Delta\phi = 0°$$

$$\Delta\phi = 90°$$

$$\Delta\phi = 150°$$

$$\Delta\phi \cong 180°$$

Fig. 1-10. Summation of two sine waves with the same frequency but different phases. When the sine waves are in phase ($\Delta\phi = 0°$), their signals augment each other, producing total signal *(solid line)* with twice the amplitude of the individual waves *(dotted lines)*. As $\Delta\phi \to 180°$ (out-of-phase condition), the two waves destructively interfere, yielding a net signal approaching zero..

To understand the more complex aspects of frequency and phase encoding of the MR image, therefore, it is first necessary to know what happens when two sine waves are added together. If two sine waves have the same frequency but different phases, their summation is another sine wave with the same base frequency but a different amplitude and phase. When the two waves are perfectly in phase with each other, their signals augment each other (Fig. 1-10). When they are slightly out of phase with each other, the overall signal is diminished, and they are said to destructively interfere. When the phase shift between them reaches 180°, the two waves exactly cancel each other.

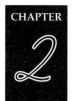
Introduction to Nuclear Magnetic Resonance

In this chapter I answer questions concerning the origin and nature of the nuclear magnetic resonance (NMR) phenomenon. Although this material seems difficult, please do not be discouraged by it. Many students get so bogged down trying to visualize what is happening to *individual* protons at the subatomic level that they often lose sight of the bigger picture. Moreover, this confusion may prove so frustrating that the student abandons all attempts to understand other aspects of MR physics. Don't let this happen to you!

I believe part of the problem is that many textbooks juxtapose and mix two different physical explanations for NMR: (1) the *classical model*, with tiny bar magnets spinning similar to tops, subject to the laws of classical physics and electromagnetism, and (2) the *quantum mechanical model*, with spin states, discrete energy levels, and the like, which are subject to a different set of nonintuitive rules that subatomic particles must obey.

A few subtle aspects of the NMR phenomenon can be explained adequately only by quantum mechanics, and we must either accept these by blind faith or learn enough about them so they are at least "comfortably familiar" to us. For most purposes, however, a detailed background in quantum mechanics is unnecessary for a good functional understanding of MR imaging. You may find it reassuring that only a few scientists doing MR imaging research in academics or industry use (or even remember much about) quantum mechanics in their daily work. Fortunately, the more easily understood classical model provides a solid foundation for describing how the NMR signal is generated and manipulated for imaging purposes. Moreover, in MR imaging we measure not the signal from individual nuclei, but only the averaged signal from billions and billions of nuclei contained within each small volume of tissue. When the averaged behavior of large numbers of nuclei is considered, predictions of the quantum and classical models converge, so our dependence on the classical description of NMR has a theoretical justification.

Q **2.01**	**You seem to use *NMR, MR,* and *MRI* interchangeably. Are there any differences among these terms?**

Historically, various names and abbreviations have been applied to the process of recording the stimulated absorption and emission of energy from nuclei placed within a magnetic field. In the original physics literature of the 1940s, this phenomenon was called *nuclear induction*; in the early 1950s, it was called *nuclear paramagnetic resonance*. Since the late 1950s, the term *nuclear magnetic resonance (NMR)* has been the preferred name for this same physical process.

When imaging methods using the NMR signal were first developed, the term *NMR imaging* was applied to them. At least partially because of patients' concerns over the dangers of *nuclear* energy, *nuclear* radioactivity, and the like, by the mid-1980s the word "nuclear" had been largely dropped when referring to these imaging methods. *Magnetic resonance (MR) imaging*, or simply *MRI*, became the preferred designation for this new radiological technique. Even newer additions to the MR lexicon include *MRA (magnetic resonance angiography)* and *MRS (magnetic resonance spectroscopy)*.

In current use, therefore, the term *NMR* is preferable when one is describing the physical phenomenon itself or when referring to the measurements of the nuclear induction signal in physics or chemistry laboratories. *MR* terminology is more frequently used to refer to imaging or spectroscopic techniques with people or animals as subjects. Furthermore, most radiology journals prefer to use the phrase *MR imaging* rather than MRI when referring to the clinical technique.

Reference

Axel L, Margulis AR, Baum S. Glossary of MR terms, 3rd ed. Reston, VA: American College of Radiology, 1991.

You also seem to intermix the terms *protons, nuclei,* and *spins* when referring to the NMR phenomenon. Are their connotations different?

By definition, NMR is a process involving the absorption and emission of energy by nuclei. *For clinical imaging purposes, we record signals principally from the nuclei of hydrogen.* Since the hydrogen nucleus consists of a single proton, we sometimes say the NMR signal comes from protons. This terminology is incorrect, however, if one is referring to other elements, such as ^{23}Na or ^{31}P, which also may undergo NMR. In these larger elements the NMR phenomenon is a property of the entire nucleus (i.e., protons and neutrons in the aggregate) rather than of the individual nucleons.

The term *spin* is derived from the quantum mechanical description of NMR in which each subatomic particle, including the entire nucleus, is assigned a *spin quantum number (I)*. This number, also called the *nuclear spin* or simply *spin*, is directly proportional to the particle's angular momentum and thus its ability to undergo NMR.

Nuclei with even numbers of both protons and neutrons have $I = 0$ and therefore possess no net angular momentum. These nuclei, such as ^{4}He, ^{12}C, and ^{32}S, cannot experience NMR under any conditions. Nuclei with odd numbers of both protons and neutrons have spin quantum numbers that are positive integers. Examples include ^{14}N ($I = 1$), ^{2}H (deuterium, $I = 1$), and ^{10}B ($I = 3$). All other nuclei have spins that are half integral, including ^{1}H ($I = \frac{1}{2}$), ^{17}O ($I = \frac{5}{2}$), ^{19}F ($I = \frac{1}{2}$), ^{23}Na ($I = \frac{3}{2}$), and ^{31}P ($I = \frac{1}{2}$). Throughout the entire periodic table of elements, nuclear spins ranging from $I = 0$ to $I = 7$ may be found. Surprisingly, there is no simple formula to calculate the actual value of I on the basis of the number of protons and neutrons in a nucleus.

In quantum mechanics the value of I for a particular nucleus determines the number of measurable discrete (Zeeman) energy levels for that nucleus when it is placed in an external magnetic field, $\mathbf{B_o}$. These energy levels (E_m) can be shown to be

$$E_m = -m\, \gamma\, \hbar\, B_o$$

where γ is called the *gyromagnetic ratio* (a constant specific to a particular nucleus), $\hbar$ is Planck's constant divided by 2π, B_o is the magnetic field strength, and m is a quantum number that may assume the values

$$-I, -I+1, \ldots, I-1, +I$$

There are thus $(2I + 1)$ energy levels, each separated by

$$\Delta E = \gamma \, \hbar \, B_o$$

According to Planck's law, the frequency (ω) of a photon corresponding to a quantized energy transition of size ΔE can be written

$$\Delta E = \hbar \omega$$

Combining the last two equations, we obtain

$$\omega = \gamma \, B_o$$

which is the famous Larmor relationship.

For hydrogen (with $I = \frac{1}{2}$) there are thus two Zeeman energy levels, separated by a transition frequency $\omega = \gamma B_o$. These energy levels correspond to the two principal quantized states of the proton, denoted $|\frac{1}{2}\rangle$ and $|-\frac{1}{2}\rangle$, also known as the "spin-up and spin-down" or "parallel and antiparallel" states. It should be emphasized that this nomenclature does not imply the spins can only "point" either parallel or antiparallel to the field and does not mean the spins actually "flip" from one state to the other. This statement simply reflects the observation that when we make measurements on a group of spins placed within a magnetic field, we always find that they are separated by discrete energy levels, and this separation depends linearly on the strength of the magnetic field. Thus, the higher the field is, the larger is the separation of Zeeman energies observed and the larger the transition frequency between them.

To make matters even more confusing, sometimes the word *spin* refers to the magnetic properties of a *group* of similar protons rather than those of a single proton. Here the word *spin* is an abridged form of a longer term, *spin isochromat*. A spin isochromat (literally, "spins of the same color") is a concept that allows us to discuss groups of individual spins that behave similarly. This notation is convenient because it frees us from constantly coping with the peculiarities of quantum mechanics in explaining the more general aspects of NMR and MRI. Specifically, we do not have to deal with the quantum uncertainties of a single proton, such as knowing exactly which state it is in or in precisely which direction its magnetic moment is "pointing" at a certain time. Since the spin isochromat represents not one but many identical protons, its behavior can be considered equivalent to a quantum average, or *expectation*. The spin isochromat can therefore be treated as a macroscopic magnetization that can be analyzed according to the laws of classical electromagnetism rather than the laws of quantum mechanics.

Reference

Becker ED. High resolution NMR: theory and chemical applications, 2nd ed. New York: Academic, 1980, pp 9-16.

 But *all* the textbooks show protons precessing like little tops in either spin-up or spin-down orientations. Are you saying this is wrong?

Yes! These diagrams and explanations, which pervade nearly all the popular literature on MRI, are both incomplete and misleading, since they are based on a superficial interpretation of quantum mechanical principles. Although these representations are intended to help the student visualize obscure concepts, such as quantization of nuclear spin and Zeeman splitting of energy levels, they do so at the expense of accuracy. If you are satisfied with these conventional explanations offered in textbooks, please skip to Q 2.04 because the next few paragraphs will only confuse you. If the explanations offered in traditional textbooks have not satisfied you, however, or if they have left you with more questions than answers, read on.

Over the years, some of my brighter students have sought to go beyond these simplistic explanations offered in textbooks, drawing complex arrays of spin-up and spin-down protons precessing in various phase configurations in an attempt to model more detailed features of the NMR phenomenon. I admit that it is immensely appealing to try to construct such models; I did this myself in the past and even now occasionally resort to drawing spinning tops for my students (while biting my tongue, of course!). Although straightforward and comforting, these spinning-top models depicting protons existing in only one of two orientations are fundamentally incorrect. No matter how complex one's arrays of spinning magnets become, the clever student will always be able to construct logical paradoxes exposing the models' inadequacies and inconsistencies. For example, if a proton can only point up or down, how do you make a 10° or 90° pulse? Why does the transverse magnetization immediately after a 90° pulse have exactly the same magnitude as the longitudinal magnetization immediately before the pulse? Why doesn't the radiofrequency (RF) field simply equalize the spin-up and spin-down populations? Why does continued application of the RF field cause the magnetization to rotate beyond 180° instead of simply forcing more and more protons into the spin-down state?

To answer these and similar questions, spin-up and spin-down top models simply do not suffice. It is first necessary to learn more about the true quantum mechanical description of a nuclear spin. Although this discussion is not usually presented in most radiology textbooks, I hope that my explanations point the way to the "truth," even if they do not reveal it completely or to everyone's satisfaction. At least the reader should gain some insight into the way things work in the subatomic world.

The quantum mechanical description of a subatomic particle such as the proton is based on the premise of its wave-particle duality (i.e., the proton simultaneously possesses properties of both a particle and a wave). This wavelike character is expressed in terms of the wave function, $\Psi(t)$, which is a time-dependent solution to the Schrödinger equation describing the particle's energetics, with appropriate initial conditions and boundary constraints. In general, $\Psi(t)$ contains several harmonically oscillating terms, separable into those affecting each of the particle's principal states. A hydrogen nucleus has two principal states (denoted by $|\,½\rangle$ and $|-½\rangle$), and its wave function can be written

$$\Psi(t) = a\,|\,½\rangle + b\,|-½\rangle$$

where a and b are time-dependent *quantum amplitudes* incorporating the "harmonic oscillations" for each principal state. For a single proton placed in an external magnetic field, quantum analysis reveals that the terms a and b each contain a single harmonic frequency ($\omega_o/2$ and $-\omega_o/2$, respectively), whose difference $[\omega_o/2 - (-\omega_o/2)]$ is the Larmor frequency, $\omega_o = \gamma B_o$.

Simple quantum mechanical descriptions of the NMR phenomena appearing in most radiology textbooks imply that a spin can exist in either the spin-up or the spin-down state only. This restriction is not mandated in the wave-function formulation and is actually a misinterpretation of the complete quantum theory. Similarly, it is not strictly correct to say that a spin "flips" from one pure state into the other. As we can see from our wave-function description, quantum mechanics does not require that a spin reside exclusively in one or the other of its principal states; the only requirement is that the spin exist in some *linear combination* of the two states.

Whenever we try to observe a spin physically (e.g., by measuring its energy or angular momentum), however, we always obtain a result referable to one of the two principal states, never an intermediate value.

The implication is not that the spin "exists" exclusively in one state or the other, but that our measuring process allows us to *observe* only one of the principal states on a given occasion. For a wave function with coefficients *a* and *b*, the probability of observing states $|\frac{1}{2}\rangle$ and $|-\frac{1}{2}\rangle$ can be shown to be $|a|^2$ and $|b|^2$, respectively. The wave function $\Psi(t)$ can therefore be thought of as a type of probability distribution, expressing the likelihood that a given pure state will become revealed during a measurement experiment.

When an RF field is applied at the Larmor frequency, its action on $\Psi(t)$ is to induce a "rotation" or mixing of the *a* and *b* components while preserving their total amplitudes ($|a|^2 + |b|^2$). This is the quantum mechanical explanation for why the *transverse* magnetization *after* a 90° pulse is the same as the *longitudinal* magnetization *before* the pulse. It is also the reason that this same amount of magnetization, but no more, can be rotated to 180° or any other angle in an NMR fast-passage experiment. In an odd sort of way, therefore, the RF field really does "rotate" the magnetic moment of a proton, but in a manner much more complex and beautiful than the tipping of a spinning top.

In an MR imaging experiment the signal we record is an aggregate or averaged signal from the trillion-trillion or more protons within each volume of tissue. What is important is not the wave function of a single proton, therefore, but its *expectation value* or statistical average taken over the entire ensemble. When the results of an experiment depend only on the "statistical behavior" of many quantized particles, an explanation in terms of classical (nonquantum) physics is generally possible. This is indeed the case with NMR, in which the expectation value of the magnetization may be shown to have *any* orientation to the magnetic field, ranging from parallel to antiparallel and including all values between.

One of the beauties (and perplexities) of quantum mechanics is that it combines features of both discreteness and continuity. Nowhere is this duality more evident than in trying to understand the NMR phenomenon. As I have stated several times already in this short monograph, I encourage the student to abandon thinking about individual protons and their quantum restrictions. It is not needed, it will not help you, and it will delay in your ultimate goal: a better understanding of the rest of MR imaging.

Reference

Slichter CP. Principles of magnetic resonance, 3rd ed. Berlin: Springer-Verlag, 1990, pp 16-17.

| Q 2.04 | If a system seeks to minimize its total energy level, why don't all the protons simply fall into the lower energy state? |

At temperatures close to absolute zero, we would indeed expect to find the vast majority of the spins in the lower energy state (i.e., $|a|^2 > |b|^2$ for most of the spin wave functions, as in Q 2.03). At body temperatures, however, this tendency for spins to "prefer" the lower energy level is opposed by thermal motions that tend to equalize the two energy levels. The resultant equilibrium distribution is therefore a compromise predicted by the Boltzmann distribution:

$$N^+/N^- = \exp[-\Delta E/kT]$$

where N^+ and N^- represent the number of spins one would expect to measure in the spin-up and spin-down configurations, ΔE is the difference in energy between the two states, k is the Boltzmann constant (1.38×10^{-23} joules/°K), and T is the absolute temperature in degrees Kelvin. At body temperature in a field of 1.0 tesla, this equation predicts that N^+ and N^- are nearly equal; only a small excess ($\sim 10^{-6}$) of spins can be expected to be found in the lower energy (spin-up) state when measured.

| Q 2.05 | When a group of spins is driven into higher-energy levels by action of an RF field, why don't the spins immediately release this absorbed energy and drop back into their original (lower energy) states? |

Long before the discovery of NMR, Albert Einstein developed a quantum mechanical description of the emission of energy from atomic systems. Since NMR relaxation ultimately involves a release of energy from the spin system, the Einstein formulation applies equally well to NMR. According to Einstein's analysis, emission of energy from an atomic system may be either *spontaneous* or *induced*.

Spontaneous emission of energy is a radiative process involving the release of a photon and typified by phenomena such as fluorescence and phosphorescence. Einstein showed that the probability of spontaneous emission is strongly frequency dependent (proportional to ω_o^3). In the visible region of the spectrum, $\omega_o \approx 10^{12}$ Hz, and spontaneous emission is a dominant process. In the RF range where NMR energies are found, however, $\omega_o \approx 10^6$, and so spontaneous emission becomes extremely improbable. *Virtually all energy emission in NMR must be* induced *through a direct interaction of a nucleus with its external environment.* This interaction may be through the electrical or magnetic fields generated by other nuclei, electrons, or molecules.

Q **2.06**	**Why does the RF field have to be applied exactly at the Larmor frequency to tip the net nuclear magnetization?**

The RF pulse generally used for MR imaging is in the form of a rotating magnetic field, denoted **B₁**, which is applied for a short time in the plane perpendicular to the main magnetic field (**B₀**). To tip the net nuclear magnetization (**M**), this **B₁** field must rotate precisely at the resonance (precession) frequency of the protons.

To understand why this condition of frequency matching must be met, consider the effect of **B₁** on **M** when applied at the resonance frequency. Since **B₁** is rotating around **B₀** at precisely the same rate as the spins, **B₁** appears to be a constant, static field, *from the spins' perspective*. The spins now begin a second precession, this time around **B₁**, as shown in Fig. 2-1. Because **B₁** is much smaller than **B₀**, the rate of this second precession is quite slow.

In an MR scanner the **B₁** field is produced by the head or body RF coil. The magnitude of **B₁** is only about 10 microtesla (μT), compared to the magnitude of **B₀**, which is typically 0.5 to 1.5 T. The rate of precession around **B₁** therefore is only about 500 Hz, much slower than the 15 to 64 MHz precession around **B₀**.

The angle of rotation (α) produced by the **B₁** field, also called the *RF flip angle*, is approximated by

$$\alpha = \gamma B_1 t_p$$

where t_p represents the length of time the **B₁** field is applied and γ is the gyromagnetic ratio. Thus the RF flip angle can theoretically be controlled by varying either the magnitude or the duration of the **B₁** field.

We can now see why **B₁** must be applied precisely at the precession frequency for this tipping to take place. If **B₁** were applied at any other frequency, the spins would be alternately in and out of phase with it, and no effective magnetic torque generated by **B₁** could be maintained. In quantum mechanical terms, this is equivalent to saying that the applied frequency must match the harmonic frequency of the principal wave function describing the state of that proton.

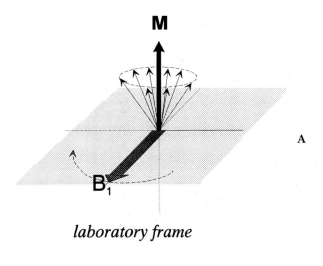

laboratory frame

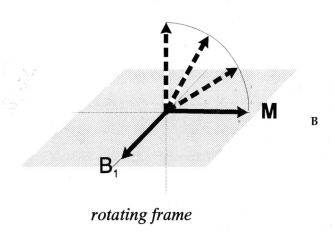

rotating frame

Fig. 2-1. A, To induce an MR signal, a second magnetic field **(B₁)** must be applied perpendicularly to the main magnetic field **(B₀)** and must rotate at the resonance radiofrequency (ω_o). In this typical representation, **B₀** and the z-axis point upward, whereas **B₁** points horizontally. Groups of spins with similar behaviors (spin isochromats) are depicted as small arrows; their sum, the net nuclear magnetization **(M)**, is a large arrow, which at equilibrium is collinear with **B₀**. When **B₁** rotates precisely at the precession frequency (ω_o), it remains locked in proper alignment with the spins so that they are all "tipped" perpendicular to **B₁**. **B,** In the "rotating frame" of reference, **B₁** acts as a constant field directed along the x-axis. **M** is then seen to precess around **B₁** in the *yz* plane with frequency γB_1.

Whereas a simple precession of **M** around $\mathbf{B_o}$ does not involve an energy exchange, the angular rotation produced by $\mathbf{B_1}$ does. Since the angle of **M** relative to $\mathbf{B_o}$ changes, system energy must also change. (Why? See Q 1.14.) Continued application of the $\mathbf{B_1}$ field results in the spin system acquiring energy as **M** goes from parallel to antiparallel relative to $\mathbf{B_o}$. With continued application of $\mathbf{B_1}$, **M** rotates beyond 180° and begins to return to alignment with $\mathbf{B_o}$. The return of **M** toward its original alignment with $\mathbf{B_o}$ requires loss of energy from the spin system. This alternate absorption and emission of energy between the spin system and the external magnetic field is another manifestation of the NMR phenomenon, further linking the classical and quantum mechanical models.

These energy considerations also help us to understand why resonance occurs only when the $\mathbf{B_1}$ field is applied precisely at the proton precessional frequency for tipping of **M** to take place. If $\mathbf{B_1}$ rotates at any other frequency, it would be alternately in and out of phase with the spins that produce **M**. In this situation, no net absorption of energy could occur. Only when the rotation rate of $\mathbf{B_1}$ precisely matches the precession frequency can **M** and $\mathbf{B_1}$ remained locked together in the appropriate relation for tipping and energy exchange. The absorption and exchange of energy constitute a resonance phenomenon, sharply tuned to the natural nuclear precession frequency.

Q

2.07

Here's *my* question to physics "experts" who may already know most of the material in this book. Does flipping the magnetization by a full 360° return the system to its original state (i.e., as it was at 0°)? How about two full rotations (720°)?

(Everyone else please skip to Q 2.08.)

The answer is "no" for a 360° rotation but "yes" for 720°! This unexpected result derives from the *spinor property* of protons. The spinor property is well known in group theory and also occurs in solid-state physics, where it is referred to as a "crystal double group."

After a rotation of 360°, the wave function (Ψ) describing the system can be shown to be identical to that existing at 0°, but with a reversal in its sign. In terms of the wave-function analysis presented in Q 2.03, this is equivalent to saying that after a 360° rotation, $a = -a(0)$ and $b = -b(0)$, where $a(0)$ and $b(0)$ were the values of a and b before the rotation. An additional 360° rotation (720° total) is required to return a and b (and thus Ψ) to their original values. Two complete rotations are required to return the system to its starting point, which can be likened to a Möbius strip, where one must travel along the strip twice to return to its origin.

I have introduced this curious spinor property to remind everyone of the beauty and complexity of the NMR phenomenon; it also provides stimulating conversation at physics cocktail parties and baffles residents at radiology rounds. The spinor phenomenon plays no role in routine MR imaging, but it *is* physically observable, having been demonstrated in several laboratory NMR experiments in which the spin-up and spin-down portions of the wave function have been ingeniously separated. Unfortunately, even a detailed knowledge of spinors will not improve one's ability to interpret MR images.

Reference

Slichter CP. Principles of magnetic resonance, 3rd ed. Berlin: Springer-Verlag, 1990, p 32.

Q **What are the Bloch equations?**

2.08

In 1946 Felix Bloch presented a mathematical formulation describing the phenomenon he called "nuclear induction" (now called NMR). His analysis resulted in a set of equations explaining the basic properties of the nuclear induction signal he had recorded.

Bloch assumed that the ensemble of spins could be represented as a net nuclear magnetization (**M**) behaving according to the laws of classic electromagnetism. If the spins constituting **M** do not interact with each other or their local environment but only with the external field (**B**), these spins experience a torque, or twisting force, given by the vector cross-product **M** × **B**. Because the torque of a system is equal to the time rate of change of its angular momentum, and because the magnetic moment is proportional to the angular momentum through the gyromagnetic ratio (γ), Bloch showed that the motion of **M** over time *(dt)* could be described by the vector equation

$$dM/dt = \gamma\,[\mathbf{M} \times \mathbf{B}]$$

When $\mathbf{B} = \mathbf{B_0}$ is constant, this equation predicts that the motion of **M** will be a simple precession around $\mathbf{B_0}$ with frequency $\omega_o = \gamma B_o$ (Fig. 2-2, *A*).

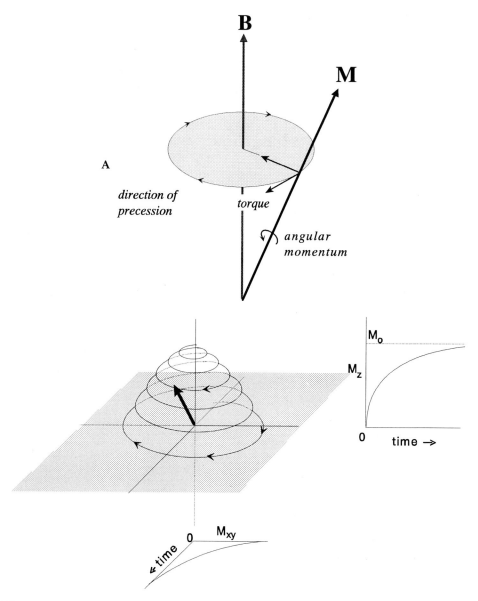

Fig. 2-2. A, The interaction between **M** and **B** is described mathematically by the vector cross-product [**M** × **B**], which is a torque, or twisting force, directed perpendicular to both **M** and **B**. This tangentially directed torque, coupled with the natural tendency for **M** to align with **B**, results in precessional motion of **M** around **B** in a clockwise direction when viewed from above. (Note that diagrams in several current MR textbooks incorrectly show the direction of precession to be counterclockwise.) **B,** Relaxation after a 90° pulse. The Bloch equations predict that **M** will spiral back upward toward its equilibrium alignment with **B₀**. Projections of this precession "beehive" in the longitudinal and transverse planes grow (or decay) with first-order kinetics, characterized by time constants T1 and T2.

If the spins interact with each other and their environment, however, **M** will not precess indefinitely around **B₀** but will seek to return to its initial alignment parallel to **B₀** with equilibrium magnitude M_o. Bloch knew that to do this, the spin system must release its energy to the environment, a process he termed *relaxation*. Bloch introduced two time constants, which he called T1 and T2, to account for the reestablishment of thermal equilibrium of the nuclear magnetization following an RF pulse. T1 described the regrowth of longitudinal magnetization (M_z), whereas T2 described the decay of the transverse components (M_x and M_y).

Bloch assumed that T1 and T2 relaxation followed first-order kinetics, such as that seen with the decay of a radioisotope. Furthermore, he assumed that single (rather than multiple) time constants were sufficient to describe this process. Another important point is that Bloch defined T1 and T2 phenomenologically and did not derive them from fundamental principles. Although he did not specify the physical mechanisms giving rise to T1 and T2, Bloch did correctly conclude that T1 must result from thermal agitation and T2 from internuclear actions. (The true atomic and molecular origins of T1 and T2 relaxation are considered in much greater detail in Q 2.09 to Q 2.14.)

Bloch then modified his original vector equation to account for T1 and T2 effects. Specifically:

$$dM_z/dt = (M_o - M_z)/T1$$
$$dM_{x,y}/dt = M_{x,y}/T2$$

The solutions to these equations after a 90° pulse are

$$M_x = e^{-t/T2}\cos \omega_o t$$
$$M_y = e^{-t/T2} \sin \omega_o t$$
$$M_z = M_o (1 - e^{-t/T1})$$

which predict that *M* will exhibit a spiraling precession around **B₀** at the Larmor frequency ($\omega_o = \gamma B_o$), as shown in Fig. 2-2,*B*. The longitudinal relaxation time (T1) therefore represents the time required for M_z to increase from 0 to $(1 - e^{-1})$, or about 63% of its final value. Similarly, the transverse relaxation time (T2) represents the time required for M_x or M_y to decay from e^{-1}, or about 37% of their maximum values (Fig. 2-3).

The Bloch equations thus arise as a straightforward consequence of a simple model of the NMR phenomenon.

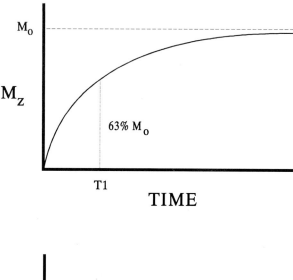

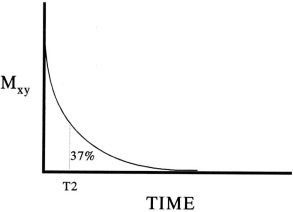

Fig. 2-3. T1 is the time for the longitudinal magnetization to regrow from 0 to $(1 - e^{-1})$, or about 63% of its final value. T2 is the time for the transverse magnetization to decay to e^{-1}, or about 37% of its initial value.

References

Bloch F. Nuclear induction. Phys Rev 70:460, 1946. (This is the original paper in which Bloch derives his famous equations. Everyone serious about NMR should at least look over this paper. It is very readable, even by those with little mathematics or physics background, and has many more words and explanations than equations. Do not be intimidated by the title or the journal. Also, you may wish to look over the next paper in this issue as well—"The nuclear induction experiment" by Bloch, Hansen, and Packard—in which NMR is "discovered.")

Roberts JD. The Bloch equations: how to have fun calculating what happens in NMR experiments with a personal computer. Concepts Magn Reson 3:27, 1991. (A version for computer hackers.)

Q | What causes T1 relaxation?

2.09

T1, the *longitudinal relaxation time*, is also known as the *thermal* or *spin-lattice relaxation time*. As previously discussed (see Q 1.13 and Q 2.08), regrowth of longitudinal relaxation requires a net transfer of energy from the nuclear spin system to its environment ("the lattice"). The term *lattice* is a holdover from early NMR studies in solids, in which the external environment was literally a crystalline lattice of molecules. Since biological NMR deals principally with liquids and tissues rather than solids, I prefer to avoid the word "lattice" and use instead either "longitudinal" or "T1 relaxation."

Because T1 relaxation requires an energy exchange, and because all NMR energy exchanges must be stimulated (see Q 2.05), *T1 relaxation can occur only when a proton encounters another magnetic field fluctuating near the Larmor frequency.* The source of this fluctuating field is typically another proton or electron, and the interaction is called a *dipole-dipole interaction.* The two spins may be on the same molecule (intramolecular dipole-dipole interaction) or on different molecules (intermolecular dipole-dipole interaction).

For a proton or electron to produce a fluctuating magnetic field, the molecule in which it resides must be moving or tumbling. To be efficient at T1 relaxation, the molecule must be rotating near the Larmor frequency. The relationship between T1 and molecular tumbling rate is represented diagrammatically in Fig. 2-4. Water, with its small molecular size, tumbles much too rapidly to be effective at T1 relaxation. T1 values are longer for free water than for any other substance in the body, approximately 4000 milliseconds (msec). When the water is in a partially bound or restricted state, however, as when it is transiently bonded to proteins and other macromolecules, its tumbling may be slowed to a rate near the Larmor frequency. The T1 value of "bound" or "structured" water is therefore much shorter than that of free water, typically about 400 to 800 msec. At the other extreme, ice has extremely long T1 values because in the crystalline state its molecular motions are much slower than the Larmor frequency. Similarly, the hydrogen protons on large macromolecules and in membrane lipids tumble very slowly and also have relatively long T1 values.

Reference

Smith H-J, Ranallo FN. A non-mathematical approach to basic MRI. Madison, Wis: Medical Physics, 1989, pp 52-72. (Gives a clear and simple explanation of T1 and T2 while skillfully avoiding discussion of the confusing spectral density function.)

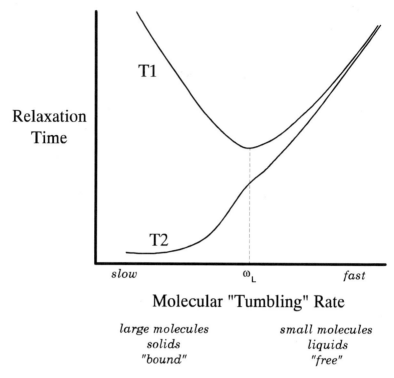

slow ω_L fast

Molecular "Tumbling" Rate

large molecules   *small molecules*
solids   *liquids*
"bound"   *"free"*

Fig. 2-4. The relationship between T1 or T2 and molecular tumbling rate.

Q
2.10

What causes T2 relaxation?

T2, the *transverse relaxation time,* is also called *spin-spin relaxation.* In contrast to T1 relaxation, where energy transfer from the spin system *must* occur, T2 relaxation may take place either with or without energy dissipation. *Anything causing T1 relaxation also causes T2 relaxation, but T2 relaxation may occur without T1 relaxation.* Therefore the numerical value of T2 is always less than or equal to T1; it is never greater. For most biological tissues, T1 values are typically 5 to 10 times longer than T2 values.

T2 relaxation results from any intrinsic process that causes the spins to lose their phase coherence in the transverse plane. Most frequently it results from static or slowly fluctuating local magnetic field variations within the tissue itself. If a spin transiently experiences a change in its local static field by a slow interaction with another spin or through an alteration in its chemical environment, that spin temporarily resonates at a slightly different frequency and thereby gains or loses phase compared with the other spins.

The terms *static* or *slowly fluctuating* include all fields produced by spins tumbling at rates significantly lower than the Larmor frequency. In practical terms, all molecules tumbling at less than several hundred kilohertz can be considered static in the NMR frame of reference, where spins normally precess at several dozen megahertz. All molecular motions in this "slow" or "quasistatic" range are therefore associated with relatively short T2 values (Fig. 2-4). In rigid molecules such as membrane phospholipids, where molecular motions are extremely slow, T2 relaxation is extraordinarily efficient, and T2 values may be as short as 5 to 10 microseconds (µsec). These extremely short T2 values cause the signal to decay so rapidly that protons in membrane lipids and most macromolecules are essentially invisible in an MR imaging experiment.

Conversely, when molecular motion is rapid, any local field inhomogeneities experienced by a proton average to zero over a short time. Consequently, these protons experience no consistent or effective static distortions in their local magnetic fields. In rapidly moving molecules, therefore, T2 relaxation processes are inefficient and T2 values are correspondingly long.

Molecular motions and interactions near the Larmor frequency may contribute to combined T1 and T2 relaxation or to T2 relaxation alone. When a proton's interaction results in the net absorption or emission of energy and a change in state, the proton loses track of its phase relationship with the other spins. Such an interaction causes both T1 and T2 relaxation. In this mechanism, T2 relaxation occurs as a consequence of T1 relaxation, and is therefore sometimes called the "T1 contribution to T2."

Two spins may also interact by "exchanging states" with each other in an energy-conserving, spin-spin interaction (Fig. 2-5). For example, if the first proton were in a pure "up" state while the second were in a pure "down" state, an interaction could occur in which the first proton flips to state "down" and the second proton flips to state "up." In this interaction, sometimes called a "flip-flop," the phases become internally scrambled, but no net absorption or emission of energy occurs. This type of interaction at the Larmor frequency contributes to T2 but not T1 relaxation and is sometimes referred to as the "secular contribution to T2."

Reference

Fullerton GD. Physiologic basis of magnetic relaxation. In Stark DD, Bradley WG Jr (eds). Magnetic resonance imaging, 2nd ed. St Louis: Mosby–Year Book, 1992, pp 88-108.

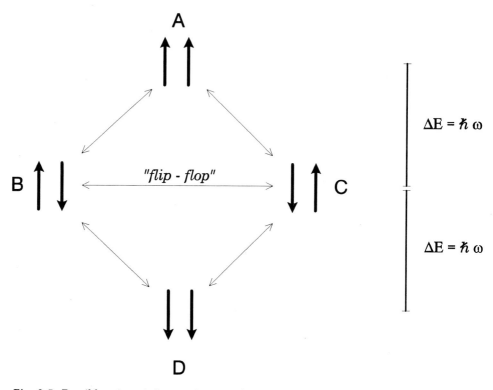

Fig. 2-5. Possible spin-spin interactions as a function of quantum states of various two-spin systems *(A, B, C, D)*. Transitions A ⇄ B, A ⇄ C, B ⇄ D, and C ⇄ D are all associated with energy exchange and thus *both* T1 and T2 relaxation. Transition B ⇄ C (sometimes called a "flip-flop") has no net energy exchange and thus contributes only to T2 relaxation.

Q 2.11	How do T1 and T2 values vary as a function of field strength?

For protons in highly mobile molecules (e.g., free water), changing field strength (and thus the Larmor frequency) does not appreciably alter the fraction of protons moving at this frequency. Thus, neither T1 nor T2 is much affected, at least over the range of fields used for MR imaging.

For protons in molecules with intermediate or low mobility, however, shifting the magnetic field to a higher value may significantly decrease the fraction of these protons able to interact at the new (higher) Larmor frequency. As a result, T1 will increase as field strength increases. For most biological tissues, empirical measurements suggest that T1 increases approximately as $B_o^{1/3}$. Therefore, measured T1 values of most tissues are approximately doubled as field strength is raised from 0.15 T to 1.5 T.

T2 relaxation resulting from static or slowly fluctuating fields is not much affected by a shift of the Larmor frequency. T2 relaxation in intermediate-mobility and low-mobility protons accompanying T1 relaxation is somewhat prolonged by an increase in field strength, paralleling the lengthening of T1. On the other hand, some mechanisms of T2 relaxation (e.g., chemical exchange) may actually be more efficient at higher fields and therefore may cause a reduction in T2 values. The net result is that T2 remains unchanged or decreases only slightly for most tissues over the range of field strengths used in MR imaging.

References

Bottomley PA, Foster TH, Argersinger RE et al. A review of normal tissue hydrogen relaxation times and relaxation mechanisms from 1-100 MHz: dependence on tissue type, NMR frequency, temperature, species, excision, and age. Med Phys 11:425, 1984.

Johnson GA, Herfkens RJ, Brown MA. Tissue relaxation time: in vivo field dependence. Radiology 156:805, 1985.

Q
2.12

What is the difference between T2 and T2*?

In the preceding questions, T2 was used as a measurement of those processes contributing to the transverse decay of the MR signal that arise from natural interactions at the atomic and molecular levels within the tissue or substance of interest. In any real NMR experiment, however, the transverse magnetization decays much faster; this rate is denoted T2* ("T2-star"). T2* can be considered an "observed" or "effective" T2, whereas the other T2 can be considered the "natural" or "true" T2 of the tissue being imaged.

T2* results principally from inhomogeneities in the main magnetic field. These inhomogeneities may be the result of intrinsic defects in the magnet itself or of susceptibility-induced field distortions produced by the tissue or other materials placed within the field (see Q 1.06 to Q 1.10 for discussions of susceptibility effects).

If one makes a certain assumption about the line shapes contributed by these processes (i.e., that they are "Lorentzian"; see Q 4.01), one may write

$$\frac{1}{T2^*} = \frac{1}{T2} + \frac{1}{T2_i}$$

where $1/T2_i$ is the relaxation rate contribution attributable to field inhomogeneities.

Q 2.13 | **How can you predict the T1 and T2 values of different tissues?**

At present, no comprehensive theory allows one to predict reliably the exact T1 and T2 values of different tissues. Sophisticated theories have been developed that adequately explain the relaxation properties of simple solutions and homogeneous preparations of macromolecules. However, tissues are extraordinarily complex, containing a wide variety of different molecules and possessing structure at both the microscopic and the macroscopic levels. Even water is not simple to analyze in tissues; it may exist in multiple states, ranging from free (unbound) to partially structured to fully bound.

The relaxation properties of most tissues can be explained in terms of two-compartment or three-compartment models, after various assumptions are made regarding exchange rates, water fractions, and the like. One such model is illustrated in Fig. 2-6, but many equivalent ones could also be created. It should be kept in mind that all such models are only crude approximations of "reality." Nevertheless, they may contribute to our understanding of basic relaxation properties of relevant tissues.

To predict the relative T1 and T2 values of different tissues and to explain their general appearance at MR imaging, it must first be decided whether the observed signal comes principally from lipid or water protons. For most tissues, water protons generate most (if not all) of the MR signal. In fact, both T1 and T2 values correlate most powerfully and simply with the bulk water content of a tissue. As a rule, the "squishier" or "juicier" a tissue, the longer will be its T1 and T2 values. For example, this principle may be used to predict and remember that the T1 and T2 values of the renal medulla (where the urine collects) are longer than those of the renal cortex, that the spleen (with more blood) has longer T1 and T2 than the liver, and so forth. Although this "squishiness" concept should be considered purely a mnemonic device and one for which exceptions can easily be found, it has nevertheless served me well over the last several years. Using this crude concept as a starting point, I was able to show (after rigorous, double-blind, radiological-pathological correlation) why some meningiomas are dark and others are bright on MR images.

Although bulk water content is a strong predictor of T1 and T2 in most tissues, the contribution of aliphatic lipid protons to the MR signal must be

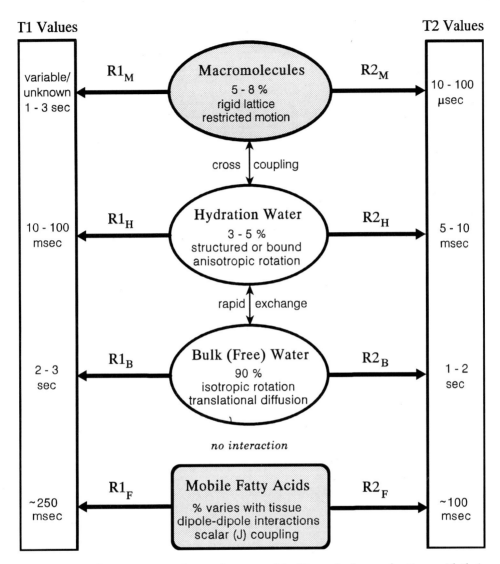

T1 Values　　　　　　　　　　　　　　　　　　　　　　　　　　**T2 Values**

variable/ unknown 1 - 3 sec	$R1_M$　**Macromolecules** 5 - 8 % rigid lattice restricted motion　$R2_M$	10 - 100 μsec
	cross coupling	
10 - 100 msec	$R1_H$　**Hydration Water** 3 - 5 % structured or bound anisotropic rotation　$R2_H$	5 - 10 msec
	rapid exchange	
2 - 3 sec	$R1_B$　**Bulk (Free) Water** 90 % isotropic rotation translational diffusion　$R2_B$	1 - 2 sec
	no interaction	
~250 msec	$R1_F$　**Mobile Fatty Acids** % varies with tissue dipole-dipole interactions scalar (J) coupling　$R2_F$	~100 msec

Fig. 2-6. A multicompartment fast-exchange model of tissue hydrogen fractions with their associated relaxation rates, $R1_i$ and $R2_i$. Many equivalent models can be constructed.

considered in other tissues. These nonpolar storage fats have short T1 values but relatively long T2 values; since they are intermediate in size, their motions are close to the Larmor frequency, and there are few static contributions to allow T2 dephasing. In adipose tissue, for example, nearly all the MR signal arises from such lipid protons. In other tissues, such as bone marrow, liver, and skeletal muscle, fat and water protons each make significant contributions to the total signal and net relaxation times. In such tissues, careful measurements actually reveal multicomponent contributions to both T1 and T2.

References

Elster AD. Magnetic resonance imaging: a reference guide and atlas. Philadelphia: Lippincott, 1986, pp 23-27.

Elster AD, Challa V, Gilbert T et al. Meningiomas: MR and histopathologic features. Radiology 170:857, 1989.

Q 2.14	**Can you explain dipole-dipole interactions a little more completely?**

As discussed in Q 1.11, the local magnetic field produced by a proton or an electron can be considered to act as a tiny bar magnet, conceptualized in the designation *magnetic dipole* (Fig. 2-7, *A*). A dipole-dipole interaction therefore merely refers to the magnetic interaction between two protons or a proton and an electron. When the interaction occurs between two protons, it is called a proton-proton dipole-dipole interaction; when it occurs between a proton and electron, it is referred to as a proton-electron dipole-dipole interaction. For either type of interaction, the spins may be on the same molecule (intramolecular) or on different molecules (intermolecular). Dipole-dipole interactions constitute the most important mechanism for both T1 and T2 relaxation in tissues.

The mathematical theory underlying dipole-dipole interactions was originally derived by Bloembergen, Purcell, and Pound and later generalized by Solomon and Morgan. This analysis reveals that the dipole-dipole interaction depends on the distance, angle, and relative motion of the two spins involved.

First, the strength of the interaction depends strongly and inversely on the distance between the nuclei ($\propto 1/r^6$). Thus, when r exceeds 2 to 3 angstroms (Å), dipole-dipole interactions are generally too weak to be detected. In large molecules, therefore, only neighboring nuclei usually affect each other. Similarly, intermolecular dipole-dipole interactions can only occur when the two molecules approach within 2 to 3 Å.

The relative orientation of the two spins in the dipole-dipole interaction is also important. To illustrate, let us consider the intramolecular dipole-

dipole interactions in a water molecule where one hydrogen proton is assumed to be stationary and the other is allowed to rotate around it (Fig. 2-7, *B*). Depending on the orientation of the two protons relative to $\mathbf{B_o}$, the field of the first proton may either augment or oppose the field of the second. Here the fluctuating field can be as high as ±7 gauss (G). The strength of the interaction between the two spins can be shown to depend on the quantity $(3 \cos^2\Theta - 1)$, where Θ is the angle between them. This leads to the interesting property that the dipole-dipole interaction vanishes when $\Theta \approx 54.7°$, the *magic angle*, which makes the term $(3 \cos^2\Theta - 1) = 0$. This phenomenon has been used to explain why certain tendons may have paradoxically low signal on routine musculoskeletal MR imaging if they make an angle of 54.7° with the field. The effect of molecular tumbling rate on T1 and T2 has been previously described (see Q 2.09 and Q 2.10). The sophisticated analysis of Bloembergen et al. justifies these results on a quantum mechanical basis.

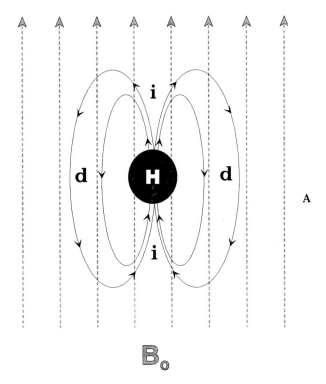

Fig. 2-7. Dipolar interactions of hydrogen nuclei. **A,** Single hydrogen nucleus *(H)* in an external field $\mathbf{B_o}$ has associated nuclear field lines around it. The net local field is increased at locations labeled *i* and decreased at sites labeled *d*. The difference in local field between *i* and *d* can be as large as 7 to 10 gauss (G).

Continued.

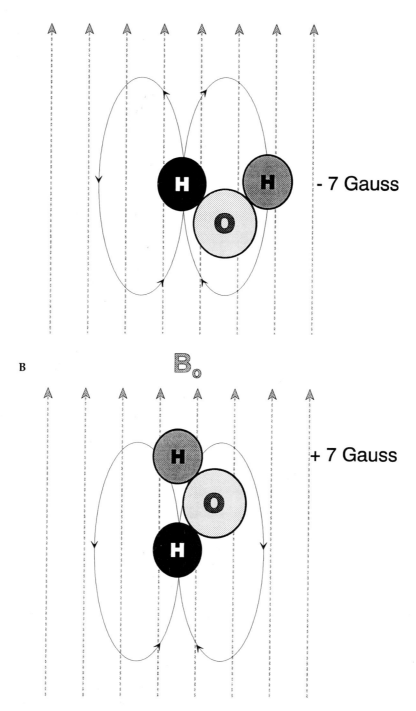

Fig. 2-7 (continued). **B,** Intramolecular dipole-dipole interactions in a water molecule *(HOH).* Let the water molecule rotate around the black hydrogen as shown in the diagram. The gray hydrogen experiences a fluctuating local field of about ±7 G as it moves between the *i* and *d* positions.

References

Erickson SJ, Cox IH, Hyde JS et al. Effect of tendon orientation on MR imaging signal intensity: a manifestation of the "magic angle" phenomenon. Radiology 181:389, 1991.

Fullerton GD. Physiologic basis of magnetic relaxation. In Stark DD, Bradley WG Jr (eds). Magnetic resonance imaging, 2nd ed. St Louis: Mosby–Year Book, 1992, pp 88-108.

Q	**What are the other important atomic interaction mechanisms contributing to T1 and T2?**

Although simple dipole-dipole interactions are the most important of all the atomic and molecular processes contributing to T1 and T2 in MR imaging, a variety of other mechanisms may be important in certain tissues and for certain nuclei other than hydrogen.

1. *Scalar (J-) coupling.* This term refers to the interaction of two nuclear spins on the same molecule by means of distortions in their electron clouds. (By comparison, dipole-dipole interactions occur via the action of electromagnetic fields "through space.") J-coupling interactions are responsible for fine-line splitting (doublets, multiplets) seen in the high-resolution NMR of chemical compounds. Although this fine splitting cannot be directly measured in a clinical MR scanner, J-coupling indirectly modulates the MR signal from triglycerides and other macromolecules, a phenomenon most prominent when the echo time (TE) is longer than 30 msec. The effect of J-coupling interactions on signal intensity in fast spin echo imaging is considered in Q 9.19.

2. *Chemical exchange.* Hydrogen atoms are frequently involved in chemical exchange processes, in which the atoms are physically transferred from one molecule to another. Alternatively, the hydrogen proton may undergo a "chemical exchange equivalent" by residing on a molecule that changes its structure or moves between chemically different compartments in a tissue (e.g., from inside to outside of a cell). Relaxation rates produced by chemical exchange processes are proportional to the square of the applied magnetic field.

3. *Cross-relaxation.* Cross-relaxation is a special form of dipole-dipole interaction in which a proton on one molecule transfers its spin to that on another molecule in the absence of a frank chemical exchange. This process may take place between unlike nuclei (e.g., ^1H and ^{15}N) or between like nuclei on different molecules. In biological tissues, dipolar cross-relaxation occurs when water molecules are closely associated with proteins and

other macromolecules. The macromolecule may act as a relaxation "sink" for the water proton, thereby facilitating its relaxation.

4. *Diffusion.* If a proton moves by diffusion throughout the course of an MR imaging experiment, it experiences an unrecoverable phase shift as it travels through intrinsic and extrinsic magnetic field gradients. This is a pure T2 effect that is proportional to the square of the gradient field and to the third power of the length of time the spin moves within that gradient. This phenomenon underlies the new MR technique of diffusion imaging (see Q 9.15).

5. *Chemical shift anisotropy.* The angular dependence of the dipole-dipole interaction is discussed in Q 2.14, as is the special case of the magic angle phenomenon. Substantial evidence suggests that the motion of hydration water associated with globular proteins is also anisotropic. This anisotropy means that the static fields experienced by the water protons may be larger and more variable than when the water is less structured. This phenomenon may explain the paradoxically shorter T2 values observed in biological tissues than would be predicted from their molecular rotation rates alone.

6. *Quadrupole-electrical field interaction.* Hydrogen does not relax by this mechanism, but quadrupolar relaxation is the most important determinant of T1 and T2 for certain nuclei (e.g., ^{23}Na) that have spin quantum numbers $I \geq 1$ and thus a nonspherical charge distribution (quadrupolar moment). Interaction with an electrical rather than a magnetic field of another nucleus causes unequal splitting of the quadrupolar energy levels. This mechanism explains the extremely short relaxation times of ^{23}Na (15 to 25 msec).

7. *Other mechanisms.* A variety of other interesting relaxation mechanisms has been described in the NMR literature. In gases, spin-rotation interactions may predominate. Relaxation in metals takes place primarily by interactions between nuclei and delocalized conduction electrons. Certain nuclei (e.g., ^{13}C, ^{19}F) relax by exchanging their spins with ^{1}H; this process is known as *heteronuclear coupling.*

Reference

Fullerton GD. Physiologic basis of magnetic relaxation. In Stark DD, Bradley WG Jr (eds). Magnetic resonance imaging, 2nd ed. St Louis: Mosby–Year Book, 1992, pp 88-108.

Q	**What is meant by a chemical shift?**
2.16	

The resonance frequency of a nucleus is determined not by the strength of the externally applied magnetic field, but rather by the *local* field experienced by the nucleus at the atomic level. All hydrogen protons within a patient therefore do not resonate at precisely the same frequency; differences in resonance frequency of a few hundred hertz exist, depending on the nature of the molecule in which the protons reside.

Placing a molecule in a magnetic field causes its electrons to circulate. In circulating, these electrons generate secondary *induced* magnetic fields. Circulation of electrons about the proton itself always induces a field that opposes the applied field. This process diminishes the local field experienced by the proton, and the proton is said to be *shielded*. Conversely, circulation of electrons around nearby nuclei generates fields that may either oppose or reinforce the proton's local field. If this induced field opposes the applied field, the proton is shielded, as before. If the induced field reinforces the applied field, however, the local field experienced by the proton is augmented, and the proton is said to be *deshielded*. When a shielded and a deshielded proton are placed within the same external field, the shielded one experiences a lower local effective field and therefore has a lower resonance frequency than the deshielded proton. Such differences in NMR absorption frequencies, arising from shielding and deshielding effects by electrons, are known as *chemical shifts*.

Q	**How are chemical shifts measured?**
2.17	

Because electronic shielding and deshielding are caused by *induced* secondary fields, the magnitude of the chemical shift is proportional to the strength of the externally applied field. If the chemical shift is expressed as a fraction of the applied field (i.e., the observed shift divided by the particular radiofrequency used), the chemical shift has a constant value that is independent of the radiofrequency and the magnetic field employed. Chemical shifts expressed in this more convenient notation therefore have units of parts per million (ppm).

For organic chemicals, the reference point from which chemical shifts are usually measured is the signal of tetramethylsilane, $Si(CH_3)_4$. Tetramethylsilane, also called TMS, is a convenient standard because silicon has low electronegativity, and the shielding of protons in this compound is greater than in most other organic molecules. Consequently, NMR signals of most other molecules are shifted in the same direction downfield from TMS. On the frequently used delta (δ) scale, TMS is assigned a value of 0.0 ppm, and most other organic molecules have chemical shifts between 0 and 10. For example, water has a chemical shift of 4.7 ppm, whereas most aliphatic lipids have chemical shifts of about 1.2 ppm.

Water and fat protons therefore vary in frequency by (4.7 − 1.2), or 3.5 ppm. In a 1.5 T scanner operating at 64 MHz, the two protons differ in resonance frequency by

$$\Delta f = (64 \text{ MHz})(3.5 \text{ ppm}) = (64 \times 10^6 \text{ Hz})(3.5 \times 10^{-6}) = 224 \text{ Hz}$$

Since the water protons have a greater chemical shift (i.e., are more deshielded), they experience a higher local effective field than the lipid protons and therefore resonate at a higher frequency. Because the chemical shift is measured in ppm, it is easy to calculate the actual frequency shift at other fields. For example, at 0.15 T with a resonance frequency of 6.4 MHz, the frequency difference between fat and water is only 22.4 Hz.

Q 2.18	How can one predict the chemical shift based on a molecule's chemical structure?

This is a difficult task perhaps best left to chemists. Nevertheless, one can reasonably understand the relative positions occupied by the common organic compounds encountered in clinical MR hydrogen spectroscopy.

Most aliphatic protons, such as those contained in fat (triglycerides), are covalently bonded to carbon atoms in relatively long chains (16 to 20 atoms). Carbon is only weakly electronegative, and the covalently bonded −(CH$_2$)− groups possess electron clouds that effectively shield the protons from externally applied fields. Most aliphatic lipids therefore have chemical shifts not too far removed from TMS, usually in the δ = 1.0 to 1.5 range.

Water protons, conversely, are bonded to highly electronegative oxygen atoms. The electron cloud in the HOH molecule is pulled toward the oxygen atom, and the hydrogen protons are deshielded (Fig. 2-8). Accordingly, these protons sense an effectively higher field than those of TMS or lipid, and they have a larger chemical shift. On the δ scale, pure water has a chemical shift of about 4.65 ppm.

Aromatic protons, such as those found in cholesterol and other compounds containing benzene rings, have even larger chemical shifts, in the range of 6 to 8 ppm. The reason for this large chemical shift relates to

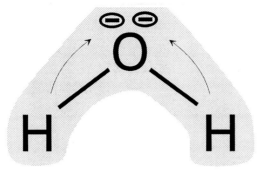

Fig. 2-8. Water protons are "deshielded" by the strongly electonegative oxygen atom, which "pulls away" their protective electron clouds.

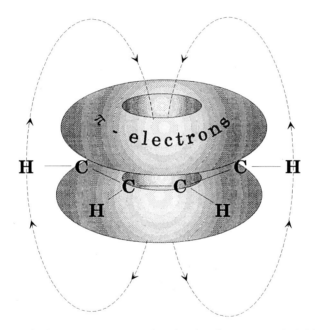

Fig. 2-9. Aromatic hydrogens experienced a localized augmented field secondary to circulating currents induced in π-electron clouds.

the circulation of the delocalized (π) electrons around the aromatic ring (Fig. 2-9). The local field induced by circulation of these electrons serves to augment the applied field, and the benzylic protons experience a local field higher than the externally applied field.

In human tissues the resonances of hydrogen protons in a variety of amino acids, proteins, and macromolecules may be recorded, but only if the strong water peak is suppressed. This is the domain of water-suppressed

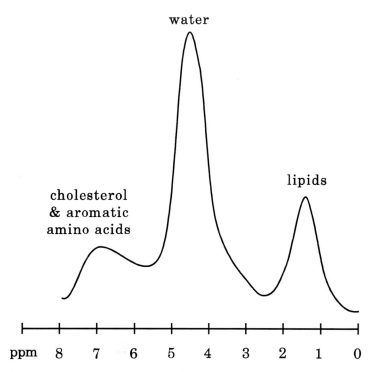

Fig. 2-10. Broad-line hydrogen spectrum through the upper abdomen of a volunteer. Most organs contain predominantly water and aliphatic lipid resonances; the liver contains an appreciable peak from cholesterol and aromatic amino acids (e.g., tryptophan, histidine).

hydrogen spectroscopy (see Q 9.08). For most imaging applications, however, the signals from these other hydrogen species are too weak to detect, and in general, only water and aliphatic lipid resonances are recorded. In scans through the liver, a moderate signal from benzylic hydrogens in cholesterol and other aromatic amino acids may also be noted (Fig. 2-10).

Q 2.19	What is a free induction decay?

Whenever a radiofrequency (RF) pulse is applied to a sample, a free induction decay (FID) signal is generated. This signal occurs because the RF pulse tips some component of the longitudinal magnetization into the transverse plane. This tipped magnetization precesses at the resonance frequency (ω_o) according to the Bloch equation formulation (see Q 2.08) and is detected by the receiver coil. The FID signal persists until the phase coherence of the spins has been completely destroyed by T2* decay. The FID signal therefore has the form of a rapidly decaying sine wave with base frequency $\omega_o = \gamma B_o$ and decay envelope $e^{-t/T2^*}$ (Fig. 2-11).

Although it is convenient to think about an FID arising from the action of a 90° pulse, an FID is created by an RF pulse of *any* flip angle because *some* component of longitudinal magnetization is always tipped into the transverse plane. (The only theoretical exception to this rule might be a 180° pulse, which in principle should only invert the longitudinal magnetization and not generate any transverse components. In practice, however, all 180° pulses are imperfect and therefore also produce FID signals.)

Q	**What is a spin echo, and how does it differ from an FID?**

In distinction to the FID, which results from the action of a *single* RF pulse, a spin echo (SE) is formed by the combined effect of *two* successive RF pulses. The first RF pulse tips part of the longitudinal magnetization into the transverse plane and generates an FID signal as before. Because of T2* decay processes, including static field inhomogeneities and chemical shifts, the FID signal rapidly dies away. If one applies a second RF pulse at time τ after the first pulse, however, the MR signal miraculously reappears (at time 2τ) as a *spin echo*. This remarkable discovery was made in 1949 by Erwin Hahn (while he was only a graduate student) and can be counted among the most important developments in the history of NMR. But where does the SE come from?

The "rebirth" of the FID signal as an SE is possible because most of the T2* processes that originally produced the decay of the FID are reversible. The FID signal has not been destroyed; it has merely become "scrambled" as its individual spins lose their phase coherence. By applying a second RF pulse, these dephased components of the original FID can be refocused into an SE. This refocusing action of the second RF pulse is usually explained using various macroscopic analogies (e.g., runners reversing their course on a racetrack, ants climbing up the edge of a flipped pancake).

In most textbooks the generation of SEs by successive 90° and 180° pulses is elaborately illustrated, and there seems little point in repeating these explanations or diagrams here. To expand your horizons, I will show you instead how a spin echo is produced by two 90° pulses! In fact, SEs will form whenever two successive RF pulses *of **any** flip angle* are employed.

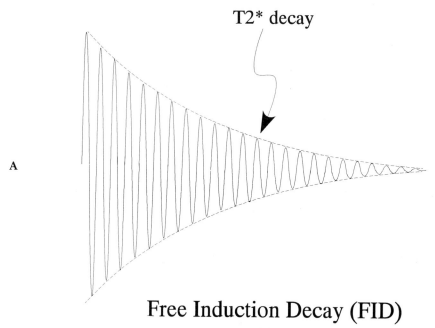

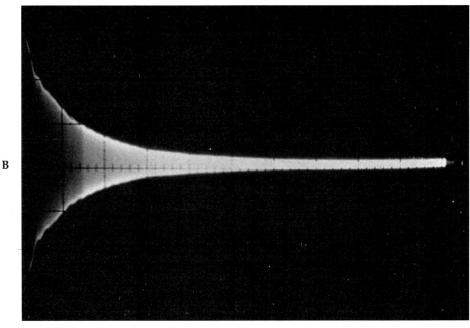

Fig. 2-11. A free induction decay (FID) signal. **A,** Diagram of an FID demonstrating oscillation at the resonance frequency (ω_o) with decay envelope of $e^{-t/T2^*}$. **B,** Oscilloscope tracing of a real FID from the author's MR scanner. Because the base frequency is 64 MHz, the individual oscillations cannot be seen, but the exponentially decaying envelope is readily apparent.

When flip angles other than 90° and 180° are used, the resultant SE is sometimes referred to as a *Hahn echo*.

Fig. 2-12 shows that after the first 90° pulse, the equilibrium magnetization **M** has been tipped entirely into the transverse (*xy*) plane. T2* dephasing causes the spin isochromats to disperse, with the fastest ones labeled *b* and the slowest labeled *a* in this diagram. The second 90° pulse then tips the entire ensemble totally into the *xz* plane. At this time, each of the spins has a vector projection along the *x* axis; the *x* components of spins *a* and *b* have been labeled a_x and b_x, respectively. (Each of the spins also has a projection along the *z* axis, a fact we ig-

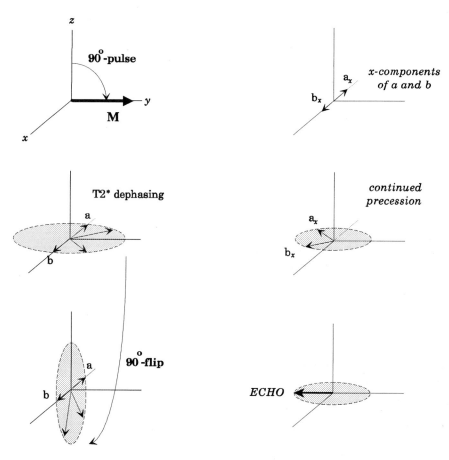

Fig. 2-12. A Hahn echo formed by two succesive 90° pulses. The magnitude of this echo is only half as large as that obtained by conventional spin echo (SE) technique (90°-180°-echo) because only the *x*-components of magnetization are refocused by the second 90° pulse.

nore for now but reconsider in Q 2.24 in our discussion of stimulated echoes.)

These "magnetization gymnastics" have not altered the intrinsic properties of the isochromats. Specifically, the spins continue to precess in the transverse plane with the same sense and speed as before. In particular, their x components (a_x and b_x) precess in the transverse plane and eventually refocus into an echo along the $-y$ axis. This so-called Hahn echo produced by two successive 90° pulses is identical to the "conventional SE" formed by a pair of 90°-180° pulses, except that its amplitude is only one-half as large. In general, if the first RF pulse has flip angle α_1 and the second has flip angle α_2, the maximum signal intensity of the Hahn echo will be smaller than the conventional SE (90°-180°-echo) by a factor of $\{\sin \alpha_1 \sin^2(\alpha_2/2)\}$.

Q 2.21 **If the SE is able to recover components of the FID lost by field inhomogeneities, why doesn't it correct for T2 decay as well?**

The second RF pulse in an SE sequence is only capable of recovering a portion of the dephased/scrambled FID signal. Specifically, the SE technique rephases only those spins whose local magnetic field does not change in the interval between RF excitation and echo formation. This condition is met only for *stationary* spins that experience *static local field distortions* (e.g., gross inhomogeneity of $\mathbf{B_o}$, a constant or symmetrically applied imaging gradient, a chemical shift, or static susceptibility gradient).

The condition for perfect RF refocusing of the FID into an SE is not met if the local field distortion changes, if the spin moves into a different part of the field, or if the spin enters a new chemical environment during the course of the imaging experiment. For example, if a water molecule diffuses within a static susceptibility gradient during the interpulse interval, its local field changes and its signal will not refocus perfectly. On the other hand, a stationary proton in a static susceptibility gradient will experience a constant field distortion that will be corrected for by the RF spin flip and refocus into an SE.

True T2 decay processes (such as spin-spin and spin-lattice interactions) occur because of time-dependent changes in the local magnetic field sensed by each proton. Accordingly, spins experiencing true T2 interactions have a random dispersal of their phases that are unrecoverable by a simple RF flip.

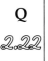

Q **Textbook diagrams illustrating the SE sequence usually show the 180° pulse flipping the spins over the top of the right side of the transverse plane. Why don't the spins flip 180° in another direction, for example, below the transverse plane and to the left?**

Small technical points such as this frequently bewilder the beginning student but are seldom explained in textbooks on clinical MR imaging. Indeed, both types of 180° flipping are possible; which type of flip occurs in a given situation depends on the phase of the transmitted RF pulse (Fig. 2-13).

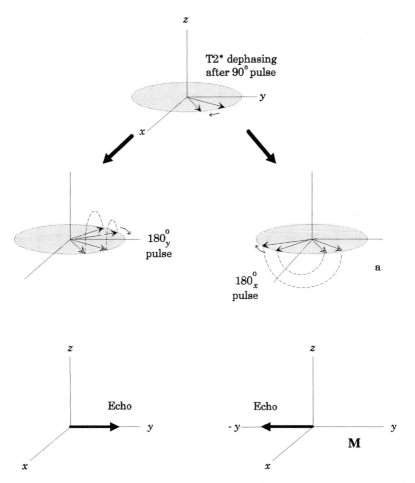

Fig. 2-13. The 180° pulse may be applied along either the *x* axis or the *y* axis, resulting in different possible diagrams and direction of echo formation.

Recall that an "RF pulse" is merely a magnetic field ($\mathbf{B_1}$) of short duration rotating at the Larmor frequency in the transverse plane. MR diagrams drawn in the "rotating frame of reference" depict both precessing spins and the $\mathbf{B_1}$ field as stationary (see Q 2.06 and Fig. 2-1). Depending on its phase relative to the rotating frame, $\mathbf{B_1}$ may be considered to be "directed" along the x-axis or y-axis (or anywhere else in between). A 180° pulse applied when $\mathbf{B_1}$ is directed along the rotating frame's y-axis is denoted 180_y° and flips the spins over the top of the transverse plane on the right side, as illustrated in many textbooks. However, applying $\mathbf{B_1}$ along x makes the x-direction the axis of symmetry; the spins flip in a different direction to mirror image locations across the xz-plane. For the 180_y° pulse, the echo forms along the $+y$-axis. When a 180_x° is employed, refocusing is along the $-y$-axis.

In the early SE experiments by Hahn (1950) and Carr and Purcell (1954), RF pulses were all applied along the same axis, usually x. In practice, this method usually results in measured T2 values that are too short because of (1) cumulative phase errors from repetitive imperfect 180° pulses and (2) $\mathbf{B_1}$ inhomogeneity that spreads out the magnetization in a plane containing $\mathbf{B_1}$ and $\mathbf{B_0}$. In 1958 Meiboom and Gill proposed that such pulse-related errors could be reduced if the 180° pulses in a SE train were phase shifted 90° with respect to the initial 90° pulse. In other words, if the 90° pulse were applied along the x-axis, the 180° pulses would be applied along $\pm y$-axes. This technique, subsequently known by the acronym CPMG (Carr-Purcell-Meiboom-Gill), proved extremely tolerant of RF phase errors and is still employed on modern MR imagers when the SE technique is selected.

Reference

Fukushima E, Roeder SBW. Experimental pulse NMR: a nuts and bolts approach. Reading, MA: Addison-Wesley, 1981, pp 28-35.

Q 2.23   **In SE imaging, why doesn't the 180° refocusing pulse invert the longitudinal magnetization in addition to flipping over the spins in the transverse plane?**

The 180° pulse *does* flip over *both* the transverse and the longitudinal components of magnetization. However, in conventional SE imaging the 180° pulse is usually applied within a few milliseconds (specifically, at time TE/2) after the longitudinal magnetization has been *entirely* tipped

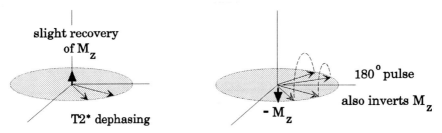

Fig. 2-14. The 180° refocusing pulse in an SE sequence also inverts the small amount of longitudinal magnetization *(M_z)* that has developed in the interpulse interval. This fact is frequently omitted from most SE diagrams for simplicity.

into the transverse plane by the 90° pulse. When the 180° pulse is applied, only a tiny amount of longitudinal magnetization has recovered that is available for inversion (Fig. 2-14). As a first approximation, therefore, the 180° pulse appears to be acting only on the transverse components of magnetization.

Q	**What is a stimulated echo?**
2.24	

Whereas an SE arises from the action of two RF pulses, a stimulated echo (STE) occurs from the action of three or more RF pulses. Let us consider the echoes produced from a series of three unequally spaced RF pulses (Fig. 2-15). These three RF pulses have miraculously produced five echoes! But from where did these echoes arise?

By inspecting the timing of each echo in Fig. 2-15, we see that echoes A, B, and C are merely conventional SEs (Hahn echoes) produced by each possible pair of RF pulses. Specifically, echo A results from pulses 1 and 2, echo B results from pulses 2 and 3, and echo C results from pulses 1 and 3. Echo D is a secondary SE produced as a reflection of echo A by pulse 3. Echo E is a stimulated echo resulting from the combined effect of all three RF pulses.

This STE results from the presence of longitudinal magnetization that has been "stored" along the z-axis by the second RF pulse. In Fig. 2-12 we considered only the x-components of the spins that subsequently refocused into the Hahn echo. However, these spins also have components along the z-axis that do not precess because they are aligned with **B**_o. During the interval between the second and third RF pulses, this magnetization regrows under action of T1 alone. The third RF pulse then flips some of this

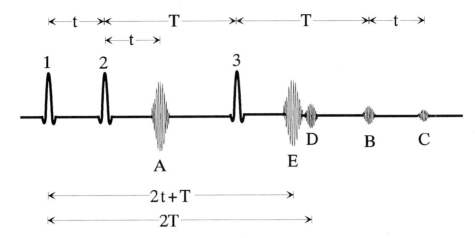

Fig. 2-15. A train of three RF pulses *(1, 2, 3)* creates three primary SEs *(A, B, C)*, one secondary SE *(D)*, and one stimulated echo (STE) *(E)*.

magnetization into the transverse plane, which reforms into an STE. The maximum amplitude of the STE can be shown to be $\{\frac{1}{2}M_o \, (\sin \alpha_1)$ $(\sin \alpha_2)(\sin \alpha_3) \exp(-2t_1/T2) \exp(-t_2/T1)\}$, where α_i is the flip angle of the ith pulse and t_1 and t_2 are the time intervals between RF pulses. If each α_i were an ideal 90° pulse and we ignore relaxation effects, we see that the maximum STE amplitude is proportional to $\frac{1}{2}M_o$. This is the other half of the signal that was "missing" when we generated a 90°-90° Hahn echo.

Some clinical sequences based on STEs have been tested and marketed (e.g., Picker's STEP). Image contrast in STE images is similar to that in conventional T2-weighted SE images, except that T1 and T2 effects are additive. Therefore, increased contrast for lesions with long T1 and T2 values may be obtained. However, because the maximum STE amplitude is only one-half that of conventional SEs, STE images are noticeably noisier.

STEs are also routinely employed in MR spectroscopy, under the acronym STEAM (stimulated echo acquisition mode). STEAM and other spectroscopic localization techniques are discussed in Q 9.07. STEs also are responsible for MR artifacts (see Q 6.13) and a significant portion of the signal generated in steady-state free precession and rapid gradient echo sequences (see Q 5.11).

Reference

Sattin W, Marcel TH, Scott KN. Exploiting the stimulated echo in nuclear magnetic resonance imaging. I. Method. J Magn Reson 64:177, 1985.

Q

Q 2.25. Are there any other types of echoes?

The only other type of echo we have not yet discussed is the gradient echo (GRE), to which the entirety of Chapter 5 is devoted. A GRE arises from the action of a single RF pulse coupled with a gradient reversal. For completeness, the four principal types of MR signals are compared in Table 2-1.

TABLE **2-1. Summary: the Four Types of MR Signal**

Type of Signal	Method of Formation
Free induction decay (FID)	1 RF pulse
Gradient echo (GRE)	1 RF pulse + gradient reversal
Spin echo (SE)	2 RF pulses
Stimulated echo (STE)	3 or more RF pulses

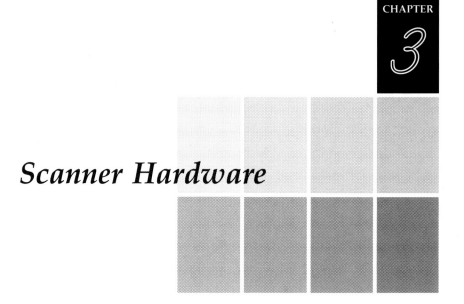

Scanner Hardware

In this chapter I discuss in more detail various aspects of the MR scanner hardware, including the magnet itself and the various coils and subsystems required for imaging.

Q
3.01

What range of magnetic field strengths are used for MR imaging? How are high-field and low-field magnets defined?

MR imagers currently available for clinical use vary in strength from 0.02 tesla (T) to 4.0 T. There are no strict definitions for "high field" and "low field," but most scanners with strengths 1.0 T or higher are classified as high field, and those with strengths up to 0.2 T are classified as low field. Scanners operating between 0.2 T and 1.0 T are usually referred to as midfield or intermediate field. The U.S. Food and Drug Administration (FDA) currently grants approval for commercial operation to scanners with field strengths of 1.5 T or less. Two companies (Instrumentarium, Toshiba) offer MR imagers operating at 0.02 T and 0.064 T, respectively; these are sometimes referred to as very-low-field or ultra-low-field scanners. Conversely, a few MR imagers with fields of 2 T to 4 T are now being manufactured and tested for clinical use; these experimental units are sometimes called ultra-high-field or super-high-field scanners.

Reference

Orrison WW Jr, Stimac GK, Stevens EA et al. Comparison of CT, low-field-strength MR imaging, and high-field-strength MR imaging. Radiology 181:121, 1991.

Q	**Are there any advantages to the lower-field MR scanners?**

Low-field and midfield MR scanners are projected to be the largest growth segment of the industry over the next several years. Cost savings of 30% to 60% compared with high-field magnets are perhaps the most important factor driving this trend, but lower-field scanners do offer certain additional unique advantages.

1. Gradient strength requirements are proportional to field strength, and a low-field magnet requires less powerful gradients for routine imaging. As a result, narrower bandwidths can be used at lower fields, with a concomitant increase in the signal-to-noise ratio (SNR). Alternatively, if gradient strength is equivalent to that used on high-field units, thinner slices or smaller fields of view can be obtained.

2. Longitudinal relaxation time (T1) is directly related to field strength and is significantly larger at higher fields. For most tissues, T1 approximately doubles in value between 0.15 T and 1.5 T. To obtain the same degree of T1 weighting, therefore, shorter repetition time (TR) values may be used at low field strengths, potentially resulting in decreased imaging time.

3. Chemical shift, susceptibility, flow, and patient motion artifacts are less obvious on low-field units than on high-field ones.

4. The fringe field is smaller around a low-field scanner. For this reason it is easier to site and shield the magnet within a hospital or imaging center. Projectile risks to patients and personnel are also reduced. Anesthesia and monitoring equipment may be brought closer to a low-field scanner.

5. Finally, low-field systems may be constructed with a vertical orientation of the main magnetic field, a configuration that offers several unique advantages with regard to coil design. Specifically, vertical-field magnets permit the use of solenoidal (wrap-around) coils, which have 1.4 times the intrinsic sensitivity of the saddle-coil design used in horizontal-field magnets.

Reference

Hoult DI, Chen CN, Sank VJ. The field dependence of NMR imaging. II. Arguments concerning an optimal field strength. Magn Reson Med 3:730, 1986.

| Q 3.03 | What disadvantages do low-field magnets have? |

Although several complex factors determine image quality, it is generally accepted that SNR is approximately proportional to field strength. All other things being equal, therefore, SNR is smaller in a low-field scanner. Consequently, to maintain equivalent SNR, more signal averages are necessary in a low-field scanner. That is, imaging time must be increased for the low-field unit.

Susceptibility effects are also proportional to field strength. Although this may be an advantage for low-field scanners because some artifacts are reduced, it may also be a disadvantage. In particular, low-field units are inferior to high-field ones in their ability to detect focal areas of calcification, iron accumulation, or hemorrhage.

Finally, because most MR manufacturers have devoted the bulk of their research and development efforts over the last decade to intermediate-field and high-field scanners, low-field units at present do not offer as wide a spectrum of pulse sequences, imaging options, and other frills available on the high-field units. This situation is rapidly changing, however, as interest becomes focused on these lower-field alternatives.

Reference

Chen CN, Sank VJ, Cohen SM, Hoult DI. The field dependence of NMR imaging. I. Laboratory assessment of signal-to-noise ratio and power deposition. Magn Reson Med 3:722, 1986.

| Q 3.04 | Is the MR magnet ever turned off? |

For most MR scanners, the answer is "no," except at times of special servicing or during installation of certain hardware upgrades. Permanent magnet systems (e.g., Hitachi MRP-5000, Toshiba Access), however, can never be shut off. Superconducting magnets (e.g., GE Signa) can be "ramped up" and "ramped down" over several hours, but this procedure must be performed under the watchful eye of an experienced service engineer to prevent sudden boil-off of cryogens (i.e., a quench; see Q 3.06). Since the electrical resistance of the superconducting field coil is zero, leaving the magnet "on" does not incur any significant costs for electrical power and allows for the maintenance of a stable, homogeneous magnetic field.

Only resistive MR scanners (e.g., Resonex RX 5000HP) are typically turned on and off at the beginning and end of each workday. These scanners can be shut down instantly by cutting off the current and can be ramped up to a full and homogeneous field in 15 to 30 minutes. Cutting off power to these magnets during times of nonuse results in a significant savings of cost and energy.

Q 3.05	How often do cryogens need to be added to a superconducting MR scanner? Approximately how much does this cost?

"Topping off" of cryogens in a modern superconducting scanner is required about every 2 weeks and should be performed as part of normal preventive maintenance by a qualified service engineer. Most scanners use both liquid nitrogen and liquid helium, but some newer models require helium only. Since liquid nitrogen is in the outermost compartment, it boils off more quickly and needs to be replenished more frequently than liquid helium. Cryogen prices vary according to service contract, locale, and vendor, but you can expect to pay about $20,000 per year for liquid helium and $15,000 per year for nitrogen on a modern 1.5 T scanner.

Q 3.06	What occurs during a magnet quench?

A quench refers to a magnet's sudden loss of superconductivity when its temperature is raised. In the superconducting state the resistance of the magnet coil windings is zero, and thus no energy is required to maintain current flow. If the coil temperature rises above the superconductivity threshold, the windings suddenly develop a finite resistance. The several dozen amperes of circulating current passing through this elevated coil resistance create heat. This heat causes a sudden, explosive boil-off of cryogens.

In my 10 years of experience with MR scanners in the clinical setting, I have witnessed three quenches. All occurred during installation or servicing when no patients were present. Generally, the only warning of an impending quench is 5 to 10 seconds of a mild hissing sound caused by a small volume of cryogens escaping through the boil-off valve. Roaring or loud hissing typically follows for about 20 to 30 seconds as great quantities of cryogens are released. If the facility is properly designed, nearly all the cryogens should escape to the outside, with a large cloud of vapors seen billowing into the sky. Generally there is also some component of cryogen escape into the scanner room as well, and in each of the cases I have witnessed, the room was also filled with a smokelike mist. One of my more vivid memories of these quenches is a marked chill in the air; the vaporized cryogens immediately cool the room by 10° to 15°.

Although gaseous helium is lighter than air and floats to the top of the room, gaseous nitrogen is much less buoyant and displaces oxygen-containing air at ground level. It should be recognized that these vapors are potentially lethal and, if inhaled, may cause loss of consciousness within 5 to 10 seconds. Continued exposure may result in hypoxia and death. Patients must therefore be evacuated immediately if a quench occurs.

Q 3.07	The MR salesperson says a magnet has a homogeneity of 1 ppm. Is this good or bad?

Most radiologists understand magnet specifications about as well as carburetor air-fuel ratios, and the vendors of poor-quality magnets prefer it this way.

The term *magnet homogeneity* simply refers to how uniform the magnetic field is when no patient occupies it. Magnetic field homogeneities are generally quoted in ppm (parts per million) of variation over a certain field of view (spherical diameter). The diameters usually specified are in the range of 20 to 50 cm. For example, in a 1.0 T magnet with a homogeneity of 1 ppm over 20 cm, no two points within 10 cm of isocenter differ by more than 0.000001 T. When evaluating a scanner's specifications, therefore, it clearly makes a difference whether the homogeneity quoted is over a 20 cm or a 50 cm range.

For MR spectroscopy measurements, it is also necessary to consider the *temporal stability* of the field. How long can the 1 ppm homogeneity be maintained? Is there drift in the field? If the spectral lines being recorded are separated by only a few parts per million, temporal instability of a magnet may ruin an experiment lasting more than a few minutes.

Before purchasing a permanent magnet, it is important to ask about the *temperature stability* of the field. If the room temperature rises by a few degrees, by how much will the field change or lose homogeneity?

The magnetic *fringe field* specification may also be important for siting purposes if space is a problem. Without additional shielding, the distance to the 5 G line usually represents the environmental limits of the magnet (i.e., how close computers or people with pacemakers may approach).

Q 3.08 | What about specifications for gradients?

Both spatial resolution and imaging speed depend on good gradient performance, and scanners differ in this specification.

The first value to look for on the specification sheet is *maximum* (or *peak*) *gradient strength*. This is usually quoted in units of millitesla per meter (mT/m). Most scanners have maximum gradient strengths of about 10 mT/m. For fast scanning and echo planar operation, gradient strengths of 20 to 40 mT/m should be sought. Concerning gradient strength, therefore, larger is better.

The rate at which this maximum gradient strength can be attained is also important. The speed of gradient ramping to full strength is called the *rise time*. For routine imaging, rise times of about 1.0 msec from 0 to 10 mT/m are good. For echo planar imaging, rise times less than 0.2 msec may be needed. Concerning gradient rise times, therefore, smaller is better.

Q 3.09 | What is shimming?

Shimming refers to adjustments made to the scanner to improve its homogeneity. Shimming may be passive or active.

Passive shimming is performed during magnet installation by literally gluing on pieces of sheet metal at certain locations, generally on the outer surface of the scanner.

Active shimming is performed by the activation of specialized coils that are adjusted to achieve maximum homogeneity. These shim coils may be resistive, superconductive, or both. Most MR spectroscopy experiments require that careful additional shimming be performed before data acquisition. This process combines manual and automated steps and usually takes 3 to 10 minutes to complete.

Q	What are eddy currents?
3.10	

Eddy currents are electrical currents induced in a conductor by a changing magnetic field. Eddy currents are generated when the imaging gradients turn on and off. These currents may be induced in the patient, in cables or wires around the patient, or in the MR magnet itself. Eddy currents induced in the patient or in wires are discussed in Chapter 10. The present discussion deals with eddy currents induced in the MR scanner itself.

Within the MR scanner, eddy currents are induced within the gradient coils, cryoshields, and radiofrequency (RF) shields. These eddy currents create various problems, impairing overall scanner performance and creating imaging artifacts. Eddy currents are particularly troublesome when gradients must be turned on and off quickly, as in rapid gradient echo imaging techniques or in MR angiography. Without compensation for eddy currents, electrical pulses sent to energize imaging gradients become distorted. These distorted gradient waveforms may produce image artifacts, including spatial blurring and misregistration. Fortunately, two methods are available to overcome the effect of eddy currents.

The first technique, used by all manufacturers, is known as preemphasis or precompensation. This method does not eliminate or reduce eddy currents but merely compensates for them. The technique involves purposely distorting the gradient-driving currents so that after eddy currents act, an output wave of the desired shape is produced (Fig. 3-1).

A second method, which actually reduces eddy currents, is to use shielded gradients. This method involves redesigning the magnet to incorporate shielding coils between the gradient coils and main windings. When the gradient coils are energized, current of opposite polarity is directed into the shielding coils. This active shield counteracts the magnetic field of the imaging gradient locally and thus effectively reduces or eliminates eddy currents.

Although shielded-gradient magnet designs seem to be gaining in popularity, certain unique problems are associated with them. Because the shielded gradients are applied in a direction opposite to that of the gradient magnetic field, they may reduce the amplitude or efficiency of the imaging gradients. Peak gradient strength, rise time, and duty cycle may be adversely affected.

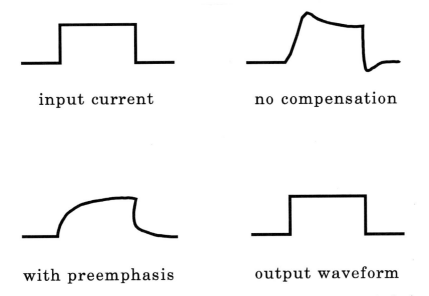

input current   no compensation

with preemphasis   output waveform

Fig. 3-1. Effect of eddy currents on gradient waveforms. If input current is in the form of rectangular pulse, gradient currents will distort the wave into the form shown as "no compensation." To correct in advance for this distorting effect of eddy currents, the input waveform is modified ("with preemphasis"). The final output waveform is now of the desired shape.

Reference

Stetter E. Instrumentation. In Edelman RR, Hesselink JR (eds). Clinical magnetic resonance imaging. Philadelphia: Saunders, 1990, pp 355-376.

Q 3.11	Is "active shielding" the same as "gradient shielding"?

No. Gradient shielding (see Q 3.10) is only one type of active shielding that may be incorporated into a magnet's design. More often, active shielding refers to the use of secondary shielding coils placed inside the cryostat but outside the windings of the main magnetic field. The purpose of these active shields is to minimize the fringe field of the scanner for siting purposes. This type of active shield has nothing to do with compensation of eddy currents.

Q 3.12	What is a quadrature coil?

The earliest transmit/receive coils for MR imaging were *linearly polarized*. In these coils, both transmission and reception of electromagnetic radiation took place along a single axis. Although easier to design, the linearly polarized arrangement was inefficient at transmitting useful RF power and was incapable of extracting all the useful information about the signal possible from the sample.

The solution to many of these limitations is to use a coil design known as *quadrature*, or *circularly polarized*. The advantage of quadrature detection is illustrated in Fig. 3-2. As this drawing shows, the true position of the magnetization in space is unequivocal only when two receivers are

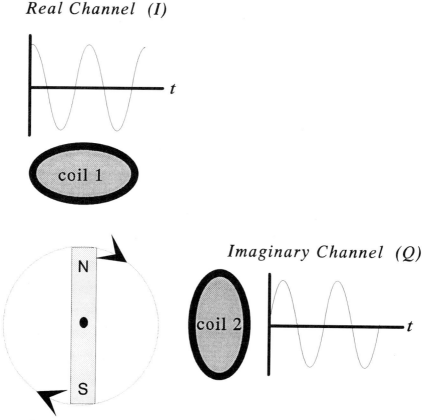

Real Channel (I)

Imaginary Channel (Q)

Fig. 3-2. Quadrature detection. Coils 1 and 2, oriented perpendicularly, detect components of the MR signal phase shifted by 90°. As the north pole of the magnet sweeps by coil 1, the signal in this channel is maximal, whereas the signal in coil 2 is zero.

present. Additionally, since two separate signals are being recorded by this system, a potential SNR gain of $\sqrt{2}$ is possible in the quadrature arrangement. Quadrature coils are also much more efficient in their transfer of RF power to the patient, reducing the specific absorption rate (SAR) requirements by one-half compared with linearly polarized coils.

Reference

Hayes CE, Edelstein WA, Schenck JF et al. An efficient, highly homogeneous radiofrequency coil for whole-body NMR imaging at 1.5 T. J Magn Reson 63:622, 1985.

Q	**What is the difference between the real and imaginary**
3.13	**channels? How can one signal be more real than another?**

The designation of MR signal channels as "real" and "imaginary" is entirely arbitrary. The signal from one channel is no more or less "real" than that from the other channel. The terms *in phase* and *in quadrature* are perhaps more appropriate than *real* and *imaginary*, and the two channels are therefore often denoted *I* and *Q*, respectively. "In phase" and "in quadrature" are defined as components of the total signal that are phase shifted 0° and 90° compared with the reference RF oscillator within the scanner, respectively.

The magnetization can thus be represented as a vector in space, with "real" and "imaginary" components recorded from the *I* and *Q* channels (Fig. 3-3.) The signal data may be reconstructed in several ways: (1) as a "real" image, (2) as an "imaginary" image, (3) as a magnitude image, or (4) as a phase image.

In Fig. 3-4, I have reconstructed the data from the real and imaginary channels separately to illustrate this process more concretely. Note that neither channel reveals the entire image completely; the horizontal bands are phase shifted from each other by 90°. For most imaging applications, magnitude-reconstructed images are obtained, computed as the square root of the sum of squares of the real and imaginary data:

$$Mag = \sqrt{Re^2 + Im^2}$$

where *Mag* is the magnitude image and *Re* and *Im* are the real and imaginary data at each point.

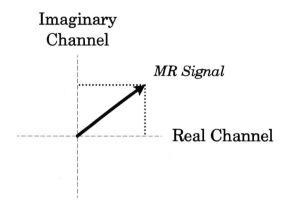

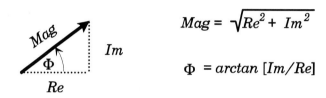

$$Mag = \sqrt{Re^2 + Im^2}$$

$$\Phi = arctan\ [Im/Re]$$

Fig. 3-3. The MR signal can be considered to be a magnetic vector with real (in phase) and imaginary (quadrature) components relative to the reference oscillator. Images may be reconstructed by magnitude or phase.

It is also possible to use the real and imaginary data to compute a phase image (Φ), where

$$tan\ \Phi = \frac{Im}{Re}$$

Phase images are occasionally useful for depiction of flow and susceptibility distortions.

| Q | What is a phased-array coil, and why is it five times more expensive than other coils? |

A phased-array coil system consists of several small independent surface coils that feed into separate receivers. The phased-array system marketed by GE Medical Systems includes six separate coils that may be combined

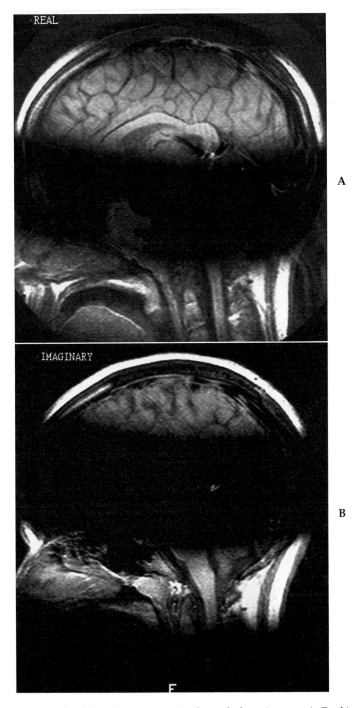

Fig. 3-4. Comparison of real, imaginary, magnitude, and phase images. **A,** Real image (data from in-phase channel, *I*). **B,** Imaginary image (data from quadrature channel, *Q*).

Continued.

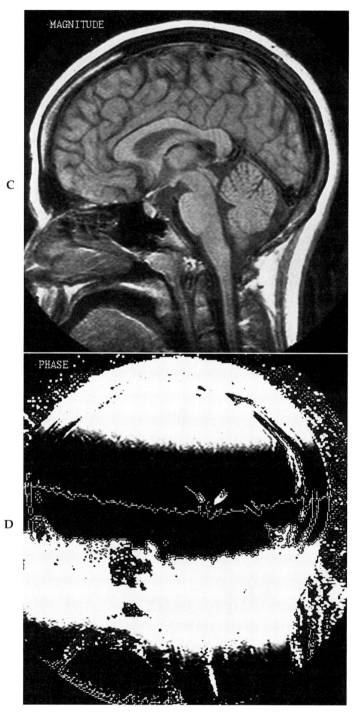

Fig. 3-4 (continued). **C,** Magnitude image (Mag). **D,** Phase image (Φ).

into both linear and three-dimensional (3D) arrangements to allow imaging of the spine, neck, heart, knee, or pelvis. Because each coil has its own preamplifier, receiver, and memory board, the noise detected by a particular receiver is limited to that transferred by a single surface coil. With this system, large field-of-view coverage (e.g., of the entire spine) can be obtained, but at a level of SNR comparable to that from a single coil and with no increase in imaging time. Interactions between the nearby coils are eliminated by overlapping adjacent coils to give zero mutual inductance and by attaching low-input impedance preamplifiers to all coils, thereby eliminating interference. The use of multiple independent receiver circuitry also accounts for the relatively steep list price of the phased-array system compared with that of conventional surface coils.

Some other manufacturers offer superficially similar coil arrays, marketed under names such as "ladder coils" or "switchable arrays." These coil arrays are not the same as a true phased-array system because only one set of receiver circuitry services all the individual coils. In these systems, only one coil may be activated at a time, but separate acquisitions may be linked together to give a picture of the entire spine without moving the patient. These switchable arrays are considerably less expensive than true phased-array systems.

Reference

Roemer PB, Edelstein WA, Hayes CE et al. The NMR phased array. Magn Reson Med 16:192, 1990.

| **Q** | **What is the scanner doing during the prescan period?** |

Before imaging can begin, the scanner must perform several calibrations to ensure its proper operation. The period when this occurs is called *prescan*. The scanner must carry out four tasks during this period:

1. Tune coils.
2. Set center frequency.
3. Adjust transmitter attenuation.
4. Adjust receiver attenuation.

The rationale underlying each of these steps is the subject of Q 3.16 to Q 3.19.

Reference

Stetter E. Instrumentation. In Edelman RR, Hesselink JR (eds). Clinical magnetic resonance imaging. Philadelphia: Saunders, 1990, pp 355-376.

Q 3.16	**Why must coil tuning be performed, and how is it done?**

Because patients vary widely in size and shape, each person changes the impedance (electronic loading) of the transmit/receive coil slightly. For optimal system performance at radiofrequencies, the impedance of this coil must be matched to the impedance of the transmission line (i.e., the wires connecting the RF amplifier and the coil). If impedance matching is not done, a large fraction of the RF power generated by the amplifier will not be transmitted into the patient as it should be but will be reflected back at the coil–transmission line interface. To ensure a good match and efficient RF power transfer, the scanner circuitry monitors the ratio of forward-to-reflected RF power while capacitors are adjusted at the coil–transmission line interface. When an impedance match is obtained, the reflected RF power is minimized.

On most modern scanners, this impedance matching is done automatically. On some older models as well as on some new low-budget brands, however, the adjustments must be made manually. Technologists must walk to the back of the scanner and adjust the coils by turning knobs or flipping switches while watching the reflected RF power level indicated by lights or on a meter. Failure to properly tune and match the coil may result in noisy images with poor contrast.

Q 3.17	**Please explain how and why the center frequency must be adjusted.**

The second step of routine prescan involves setting the center frequency. Setting the center frequency provides a fine adjustment that tells the scanner at exactly what frequency the protons of interest are resonating at magnet isocenter. (Patient-to-patient variations in susceptibility may change this value by a few dozen hertz, potentially resulting in a few millimeters of error in spatial localization.)

Setting the center frequency also allows identification and tuning on a proton species of interest. For example, the center frequency may be set on water protons, fat protons, or some average of the two. Accurate center frequency setting is particularly important when fat saturation pulses are employed.

Q 3.18	What is the purpose of the transmit attenuation adjustment?

This step in prescan, also known as pulse amplitude calibration, determines the RF output necessary to achieve a 90° (or other flip angle) pulse. Recall from Q 2.06 that the RF flip angle (α) is determined by

$$\alpha = \gamma\, B_1\, t_p$$

where t_p represents the length of time the B_1 field is applied and γ is the gyromagnetic ratio. With pulse length (t_p) fixed, the RF flip angle is controlled by varying the magnitude of the **B_1** field. The magnitude of **B_1**, in turn, is dictated by the output voltage and current of the RF amplifier. This amplifier output is scaled downward from its maximum value by means of an interposed circuit (the attenuator). The attenuator is adjusted so that the proper current and voltage are sent to the coil to generate a **B_1** field of appropriate magnitude. This attenuator setting must be adjusted for each patient empirically because variable loading of the transmitter coil alters the required amplifier output case by case.

Transmit attenuation is set automatically on all scanners, although manual overrides are possible. The scanner accomplishes this task by sending out test RF pulses at variable attenuator settings and noting the amplitude of each free induction decay (FID) signal created. When a maximum value is obtained, the attenuator is calibrated for a 90° pulse. From this, the attenuation values required for a 180° or other flip angle pulse can be calculated by simple scaling.

Q 3.19	Why is the receive attenuator adjustment necessary?

This final calibration step involves the adjustment of receiver amplifier gain with respect to the maximum MR signal occurring during imaging. If the attenuator value is set too low (i.e., receiver gain is set too high), the signal will overload the analog-to-digital converter, and data clipping will occur, causing severe image distortion (Fig 3-5). If the receive

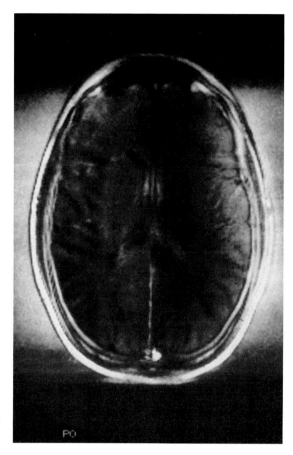

Fig. 3-5. Improper adjustment of receive attenuator (attenuator set too low). The resultant eerie image is a result of data-clipping distortion of the MR signal.

attenuator is set too high, receiver gain will be insufficient, and image noise will increase.

The scanner automatically calibrates receive attenuation by running a mock pulse sequence identical to that specified for imaging, except that the phase-encode gradient is set to zero. When the phase-encode gradient is zero, signal is maximal. After the receive attenuation is set, real scanning can begin.

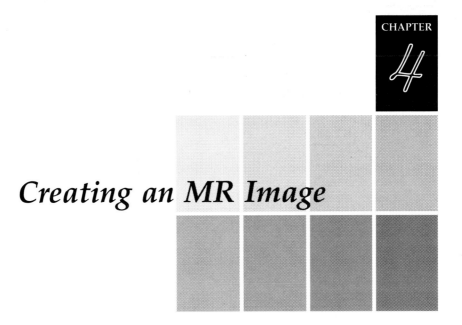

Creating an MR Image

In this chapter I answer several basic questions concerning the acquisition of MR signals and their reconstruction into the final image. These concepts are neither easily grasped nor intuitively obvious; every MR student at some time has struggled with them. Although all MR textbooks address these topics, I have found the most lucid explanation to be a monograph by Paul Keller, entitled "Basic Principles of Magnetic Resonance Imaging." This is available from GE Medical Systems as Publication 7798 and is well worth obtaining from your local sales representative, if possible.

Q	What is a Fourier transform?
4.01	

A Fourier transform (FT) is a mathematical technique that allows an MR signal to be decomposed into a sum of sine waves of different frequencies, phases, and amplitudes. In MR imaging, signals arising from each part of an imaged object are spatially encoded by differences in frequency and phase. For this reason, phase encoding and frequency encoding make the MR signal naturally amenable to analysis by Fourier techniques.

For example, consider a hypothetical NMR signal with a triangular waveform, as shown in Fig. 4-1. This wave can be approximated by summation of a number of sine waves, called harmonics, each with different amplitudes, frequencies, and phases. In mathematical terms, then, a time-varying MR signal *s(t)* can be written as

$$s(t) = a_o = a_1 sin(\omega_1 t + \phi_1) + a_2 sin(\omega_2 + \phi_2) + a_3 sin(\omega_3 + \phi_3) + \ldots$$

The Fourier series is sometimes displayed graphically, with the amplitudes (a_i) of the Fourier components plotted as a function of frequency (ω). Such a representation is known as the frequency spectrum of the signal (Fig. 4-2).

To represent any real NMR signal exactly, an infinite number of frequency components must be included in its Fourier representation. Clearly this condition cannot be met in MR imaging, since our computer memory is limited and a finite digitizing rate permits us to sample only a limited band of frequencies contained within the actual signal. The Fourier series representation of an MR image must therefore be cut short (truncated) at some point, giving rise to characteristic errors in its reconstruction (see Q 6.05).

Fourier analysis allows us to represent any time-varying signal s(t) as a spectrum of complex frequencies S(ω). The mathematical procedure interrelating s(t) and S(ω) is known as *Fourier transformation*. If s(t) is specified, S(ω) may be readily computed, and vice versa. Because the appearance of S(ω) is not immediately obvious for a given s(t), I have drawn several FT pairs in Fig. 4-3. As a general trend, when s(t) is spread

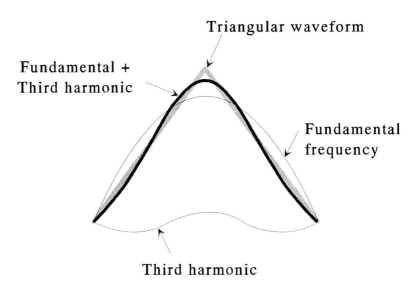

Fig. 4-1. Decomposition of a triangular waveform by Fourier methods into its principal components (harmonics).

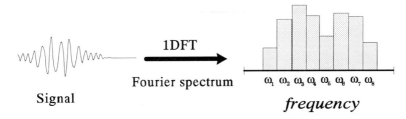

1DFT

Fourier spectrum

$\omega_1\ \omega_2\ \omega_3\ \omega_4\ \omega_5\ \omega_6\ \omega_7\ \omega_8$

Signal

frequency

Fig. 4-2. Graphical representation of the Fourier spectrum of a given signal. The height of each bar represents the relative size of the Fourier component of the signal at that harmonic frequency.

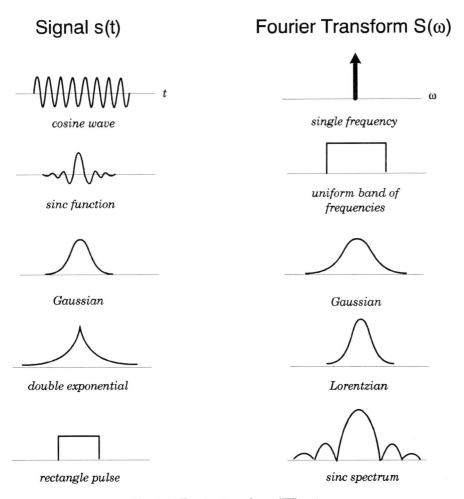

Signal s(t)

Fourier Transform S(ω)

cosine wave

single frequency

sinc function

uniform band of frequencies

Gaussian

Gaussian

double exponential

Lorentzian

rectangle pulse

sinc spectrum

Fig. 4-3. Fourier transform (FT) pairs.

out in time, $S(\omega)$ is compact, and vice versa. Note that the Fourier representation of a square wave is known as a *sinc function*, where

$$sinc(x) = \frac{sin(\pi x)}{\pi x}$$

Radiofrequency (RF) pulses are often shaped similar to modified sinc functions, since it is their purpose to stimulate uniformly a rectangular slice encoded by frequency.

Reference

Bracewell R. The Fourier transform and its applications, 2nd ed. New York: McGraw-Hill, 1986. (This classic textbook requires a knowledge of calculus but has numerous line drawings and explanations as well. Nearly all the physicists and engineers I know who work in MR own or have read this book.)

Q	How is slice-selective excitation accomplished?

4.02

Two steps are required to excite selectively a slice in two-dimensional Fourier transform (2DFT) MR imaging: (1) a slice-select gradient is imposed along an axis perpendicular to the plane of the desired slice, resulting in a linear variation of potential resonance frequencies in that direction; and (2) a specially tailored RF pulse is then applied, whose center frequency matches the Larmor frequency of the desired slice. The combination of steps 1 and 2 ensures that only protons within the chosen slice are excited.

The role of the slice-select gradient in defining slice position and thickness is illustrated in Fig. 4-4. We see that the center frequency of the RF pulse determines the location of the slice, whereas the RF bandwidth (i.e., the range of frequencies contained within the RF pulse) determines slice thickness. Alternatively, if the RF bandwidth remains constant, slice thickness may be changed by varying the strength of the slice-select gradient. These relationships may be combined into the equation

$$\Delta F = \gamma \cdot G_{ss} \cdot \Delta z$$

where ΔF is the RF bandwidth, G_{ss} is the strength of the slice-select gradient, and Δz is the slice thickness.

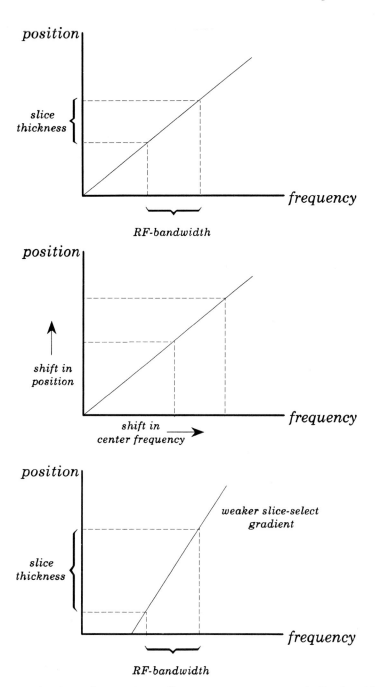

Fig. 4-4. How the slice-select gradient affects section parameters. **A,** Section thickness is determined by radiofrequency (RF) bandwidth for a given strength (slope) of the slice-select gradient. **B,** Section position is determined by center frequency of RF pulse in conjunction with gradient slope. **C,** With bandwidth held constant, weaker slice-select gradient produces a thicker slice.

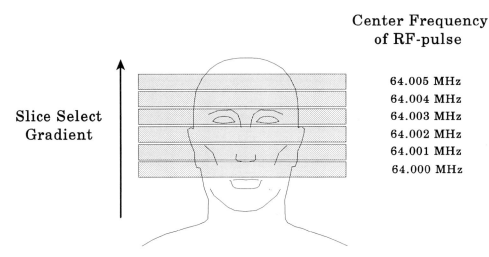

**Center Frequency
of RF-pulse**

**Slice Select
Gradient**

64.005 MHz
64.004 MHz
64.003 MHz
64.002 MHz
64.001 MHz
64.000 MHz

Fig. 4-5. Slice position is determined by center frequency of RF pulse for a given gradient strength.

By changing the center frequency of the RF pulse, we may adjust slice position. This is illustrated graphically in Fig. 4-5.

For most imaging applications, we want the edge of each slice to be as sharply defined as possible. To accomplish this goal, we must make sure that the RF pulse contains a rectangular band of frequencies whose high and low cutoff values correspond to the edges of the desired slice. As discussed in Q 4.01, an RF pulse shaped as a sinc function in the time domain produces such a uniform band of frequencies. Slice-selective RF pulses used in MR imaging often are sinc shaped (Fig. 4-6).

In summary, two steps are needed for slice-selective excitation: (1) a slice-select gradient must be activated, producing a linear dispersion of resonant frequencies perpendicular to the plane of the desired slice; and (2) the chosen slice must be selectively excited by one or more RF pulses, whose center frequency and shape correspond to the frequencies contained in the slice, as defined by the slice-select gradient.

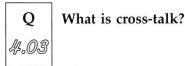

What is cross-talk?

Cross-talk refers to interference that occurs between adjacent slices in MR imaging. Cross-talk arises because time-limited RF pulses are inherently imperfect, having slice profiles that are nonrectangular.

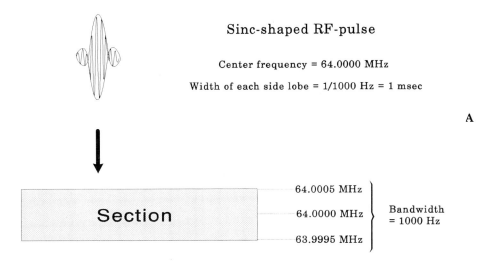

Sinc-shaped RF-pulse

Center frequency = 64.0000 MHz

Width of each side lobe = 1/1000 Hz = 1 msec

A

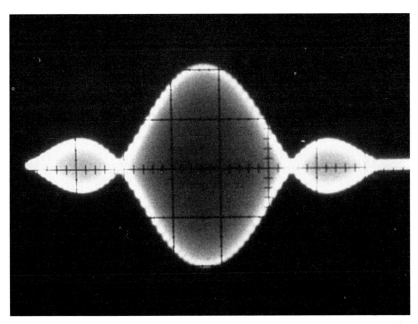

Fig. 4-6. Sinc-shaped RF pulses. **A,** Graphical representation. **B,** Oscilloscope tracing of a real sinc pulse from the author's MR scanner. Because the base frequency is 64 MHz, only the envelope of the RF pulse can be appreciated on the oscilloscope tracing.

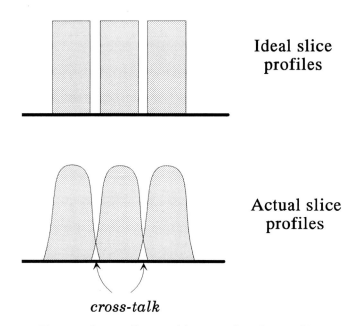

Ideal slice profiles

Actual slice profiles

cross-talk

Fig. 4-7. Cross-talk caused by imperfect slice profiles.

As discussed in Q 4.02, a perfectly rectangular slice corresponds to a rectangular band of frequencies in the slice-select direction. To excite exclusively and uniformly such a discrete band of frequencies, a sinc-shaped RF pulse with an infinite number of side lobes (and thus of infinite duration) is required. In any real imaging system, however, the sinc pulse must be shortened, and only a limited number (e.g., one to three) of side lobes can be used. This so-called apodization of the sinc pulse (literally, "cutting off its feet") results in a distortion of the slice profile, as shown in Fig. 4-7. Because the resultant slice profiles are not perfectly rectangular, they overlap at their edges when closely spaced. The RF pulses for one slice therefore stimulate protons in adjacent slices, and this phenomenon is known as *cross-talk*. Because of cross-talk, it is usually advisable to insert small gaps between slices in clinical MR imaging to improve signal-to-noise ratio (SNR) and minimize artifacts.

Q
4.04

Don't the signals from all the slices get mixed together? How does the MR scanner keep track of which signal comes from which slice?

In 2DFT imaging, each slice is individually excited and its MR signal separately recorded and stored. Multislice acquisition is possible because

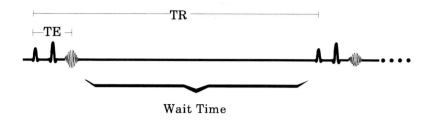

Wait Time

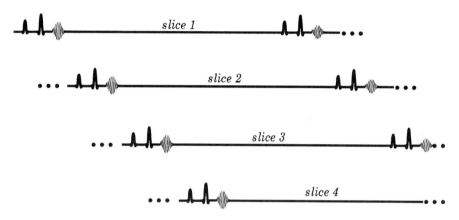

Fig. 4-8. Multisection acquisition is possible because of the "wait times" needed between echo formation and the next repetition of the RF sequence.

of the "wait times" or "dead times" within the structure of most MR imaging sequences. As shown in Fig. 4-8, the time gap between echo collection and the next 90° pulse can be put to good use by stimulating and recording signals from other slices during this period.

In three-dimensional Fourier transform (3DFT) imaging, however, slice-selective excitation is not employed. Here, slice selection is accomplished by phase-encoding methods. The principles of phase encoding are discussed in more detail later in this chapter.

| | **Q** | **How is frequency encoding accomplished?** |

Once a given slice is selectively excited, the signals arising from each volume element (voxel) within that section must be spatially encoded. In

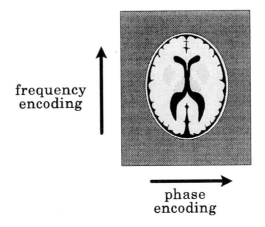

Fig. 4-9. In routine spin warp imaging, one in-plane dimension of an image is phase encoded, whereas the other is frequency encoded.

routine MR imaging, one of these in-plane dimensions is encoded by changes in frequency, whereas the other is encoded by differences in phase (Fig. 4-9). Frequency encoding is the most straightforward of the two techniques and is discussed in this section. Phase encoding is more complex and is discussed in Q 4.06 to Q 4.10.

Frequency encoding of an in-plane dimension is accomplished by turning on a gradient (called appropriately the *frequency-encoding gradient*) at two separate times during each imaging cycle (Fig. 4-10). The first application of the frequency-encoding gradient (sometimes called the *dephase lobe*) transiently changes the frequency of pixels from each column (or row) of the image according to its location within that gradient. When the gradient is turned off, spins residing in pixel columns that experienced the stronger portion of the frequency-encoding gradient have gained phase compared with spins that were in the weaker part of the gradient. The 180° pulse inverts this spatially dependent distribution of phases, just as it did in the formation of a spin echo (SE).

To refocus the MR signal into an echo, the frequency-encoding gradient must be turned on a second time (now often referred to as the *readout lobe* or *readout gradient*). Note in Fig. 4-10 that the readout lobe has twice the area of the dephase lobe, allowing the full echo to be refocused. The peak of the echo occurs at the center of the readout lobe at time TE, when complete rephasing occurs.

The strength of the frequency-encoding gradient required to encode spatially a given image depends on two operator-selected parameters: (1) the field of view (FOV) in the frequency-encode direction and (2) the receiver bandwidth (BW). The FOV is merely a linear dimension (given in

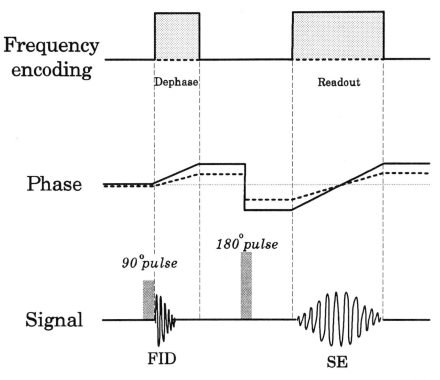

Fig. 4-10. Schematic of the action of the frequency-encoding gradient in a spin-echo (SE) pulse sequence. The first (dephase) lobe causes a phase-dispersal based on position within the gradient. The readout gradient refocuses those spins at a time coinciding with the Hahn (RF) echo.

millimeters or centimeters) selected to accommodate the anatomical region of interest. For routine clinical imaging applications, the FOV usually ranges from 15 to 35 cm. The BW represents the total frequency range (given in hertz or kilohertz) used to span the selected FOV. Typical values are 4 to 32 kHz. Note that this bandwith is the *receiver BW*, not the *RF transmitter BW* discussed in Q 4.02. Receiver BW is discussed more completely in Q 4.13.

Once the FOV and BW have been selected, the frequency-encoding gradient strength (G_f) can be computed by the relation

$$\gamma G_f = BW/FOV$$

This equation makes sense because BW/FOV is simply the defined number of hertz per centimeter in the image, and γG_f is the same, with units (Hz/gauss)(gauss/cm) = Hz/cm.

Q
4.06

How is phase encoding accomplished?

Initially it might seem impossible to determine the spatial origins of the individual MR signals produced in the 50,000+ voxels contained within a typical slice. This process is manageable, however, because the signals are acquired in an orderly fashion and linear gradients cause the frequencies and phases of the individual signals to vary predictably across the image. So far we have discussed slice selection and frequency encoding. We now turn to a more complicated topic: phase encoding of the MR image.

Before we delve into the complexities of phase encoding, it is worthwhile to reinforce one basic concept: In MR imaging, the RF pulses excite all protons in a slice simultaneously, and *a single, conglomerate echo signal is recorded from the entire slice for each phase-encode step*. This concept is illustrated schematically in Fig. 4-11, where the number of phase-encoding steps is 256; 128 positive and 128 negative gradient steps have been applied in the complete imaging sequence. Because the larger gradient steps cause more phase dispersion of the individual

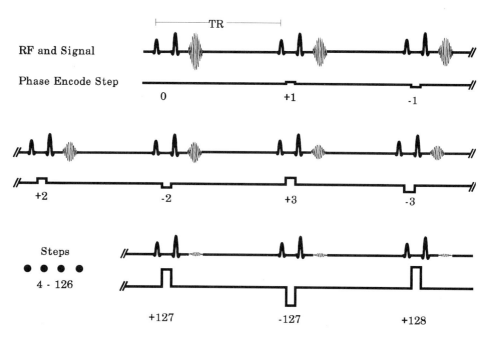

Fig. 4-11. To encode spatially a two-dimensional Fourier transform (2DFT) image, echoes must be collected for a full complement of phase-encoding steps (here, $N_p = 256$).

components, the echo amplitudes decrease as the phase-encode steps become larger.

Each step of the phase-encoding gradient produces a different amount of phase shift for each column of pixels within an image (Fig. 4-12). When no phase-encoding gradient is applied (step 0), no phase shifts are created between any of the pixel columns. After application of the first phase-encode step (step +1), a linear phase shift from 0° to 360° has been created across the image, and a shift of a few degrees now exists between adjacent pixel columns. After step +2 the phase shift across the entire image has been expanded to 720°, and the phase shift between adjacent pixels has been doubled. By the time the last step is reached, many phase cycles encompass the entire image, and adjacent pixel columns differ in phase by 180°.

The maximum strength required for the phase-encoding gradient (G_p) can be calculated from the requirement that for maximum spatial resolution, adjacent pixel columns vary in phase by 180°, or ½ cycle. (This requirement for a 180° phase shift between adjacent columns is equivalent to defining the maximum spatial resolution in terms of alternating black and white bars, as in a line-pair test pattern.) With N_p samples (pixels) in the phase-encoding direction, the maximum total phase shift across the image must therefore be ½N_p cycles, and the required phase shift per centimeter is ½N_p/FOV. If the phase-encoding gradient is applied as a rectangular pulse with maximum amplitude (G_p) for time T_p, the accumulated phase per centimeter is $\gamma G_p T_p$. This last expression, if not immediately obvious, can be verified with a unit check: $\gamma G_p T_p$ = (Hz/gauss)(gauss/cm)(sec) = cycles/cm. We now have a useful relationship for calibrating the phase-encoding gradient:

$$\gamma G_p T_p = \text{½}N_p/\text{FOV}$$

In a more general formulation where the gradient pulse may have an arbitrary shape, the quantity $G_p T_p$ is merely the area under the phase-encoding gradient lobe on a pulse sequence timing diagram. Furthermore, N_p/FOV equals 1/(pixel width), so we see that

$$(\text{Gradient area}) (\text{Pixel width}) = \text{½}\gamma = \text{Constant}$$

Pixel size in the phase-encoding direction, determined by the MR operator by selecting N_p and FOV, is calibrated internally in the scanner by adjustment of the maximum amplitude and duration of the phase-encoding gradient, according to the equations just listed.

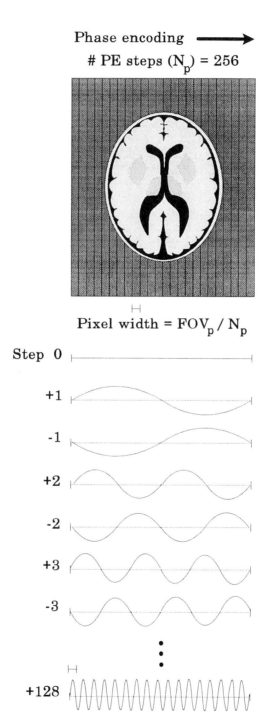

Fig. 4-12. Each application of the phase-encoding gradient produces a different amount of phase shift between signals in adjacent pixels, ranging from 0° at step 0 to 180° at step +128.

<table>
<tr><td>**Q**
4.07</td><td>**But I still don't understand how you can use phase shifts to determine from which pixel a given MR signal originated.**</td></tr>
</table>

Perhaps this issue can best be understood by means of a simple example (Fig. 4-13). Here, signals from a hypothetical six-pixel image have been spatially encoded by frequency and phase. Since there are only two rows in the phase-encoding direction, only two applications of the phase-encode gradient (producing phase shifts of 0° and 180°, respectively) are required. Two complex MR signals are thus sampled and used to reconstruct the image.

The first of these signals is acquired when no phase-encoding gradient has been applied and no phase shift occurs between the two rows. Fourier transformation of this first MR signal generates a spectrum revealing three frequencies $(\omega_1,\omega_2,\omega_3)$, whose amplitudes (A + B), (C + D), and (E + F) are

6-Pixel Image

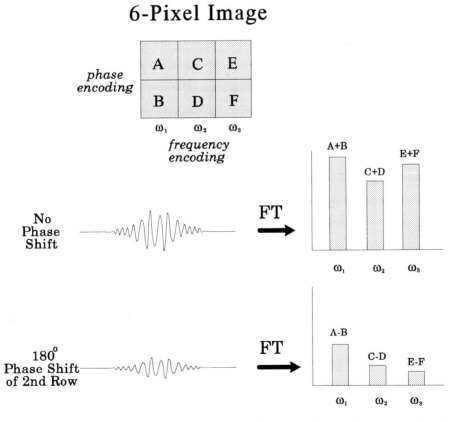

Fig. 4-13. Sample calculation showing how two phase encodings allow one to decode signals from individual pixels in a six-pixel image. (See Q 4.07 for details.)

the sum of the pixel values in each frequency column. At this stage we only know the sums of the pixel values for each frequency column; we do not know the individual values in any cell.

Now let us apply a phase-encoding gradient that leaves the phase of the pixels in the top row unchanged but shifts those in the bottom row by 180°. To see the effect of this phase shift, let us consider the summation signal from pixels A and B. If $A(t) = A \sin(\omega t)$, and if $B(t) = B \sin(\omega t + 180°) = -B \sin(\omega t)$, we see that the summation signal $A(t) + B(t) = (A - B) \sin(\omega t)$. Now when we record the MR signal from the whole sample with the second row phase shifted by 180°, the Fourier spectrum has changed. Again three frequencies are recorded, but this time their magnitudes are $(A - B)$, $(C - D)$, and $(E - F)$. We still are not able to assign unique pixel values with this single measurement, since now only the *differences* in pixel values for each frequency column are known.

When we combine the information from the first and second phase-encode steps, however, we *can* calculate individual pixel values. For example, to calculate pixel values in the ω_1 frequency column, we add the spectral amplitudes from each acquisition $[(A + B) + (A - B) = 2A]$ to compute A; we subtract them $[(A + B) - (A - B) = 2B]$ to determine B.

Q 4.08	I see how to calculate pixel values in your simple example, but how do you do this in a *real* image with thousands of pixels?

A real image is much more complex than the six-pixel example, but the general principles remain the same. Several minor differences are immediately apparent, however. First, in MR imaging we typically use 256 divisions along the frequency-encode axis, and thus the first FT spectrum has 256 frequency "bars" rather than only three. Second, the number of echo signals acquired equals the number of phase-encode steps, which is usually 128 or 256 rather than two. Third, the phase shifts between the rows are not simple multiples of 180° but vary from echo to echo depending on the size of the phase-encoding step (see Fig. 4-12). Fourth, because each echo has been acquired using a different set of interrow phase shifts, the spectral amplitudes (heights of the bars) for each echo cannot simply be added or subtracted to compute individual pixel values as before. To sort out where each signal in a frequency column has originated, a second FT must be performed.

This 2DFT encoding and reconstruction process is illustrated in Fig. 4-14. Multiple phase-encode steps generate an array of different MR signals from the phantom. The first FT of each of these signals provides a crude frequency projection of the object, modified by the phase shifts imparted

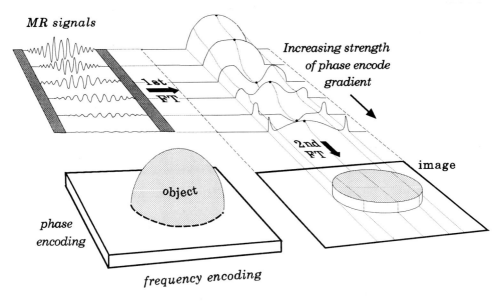

Fig. 4-14. Graphical representation of how an image section is spatially encoded during 2DFT imaging. Here the frequency encoding is horizontal and the phase-encoding direction is vertical. A set of MR signals is acquired using the same frequency-encoding gradient but different values of the phase-encoding gradient. Each of these MR signals is Fourier transformed to provide a frequency spectrum for each phase-encoding step. Each column of data from the stack of first FT "images" is transformed again to determine the spatial projection in the vertical image plane.

by each step. Note that for low-order phase encodings, the frequency projection approximates the general shape of the object but lacks edge definition. The higher-order phase-encode steps provide more information about spatial detail, such as the location of edges.

To construct the final image, a second FT is performed using data from this intermediate stage grouped into columns of the same frequency. Note that in our example, the data in each of these columns have the form of a decaying oscillation reminiscent of a sinc function. This is the case because the final projection of the object along each line in the phase encode direction is in the form of a rectangle (Fig. 4-14).

To reinforce to you that this process is "real," I have imaged a round phantom in my scanner and stopped image processing after the first FT has been performed (Fig. 4-15, *A*). Here we see that the raw signal data have been converted into a crude frequency projection of the object. Along the horizontal (frequency-encoding) axis we see the edges of the object; we are unsure at this stage of its appeearence in its vertical extent. By performing Fourier transformation along each vertically oriented frequency column,

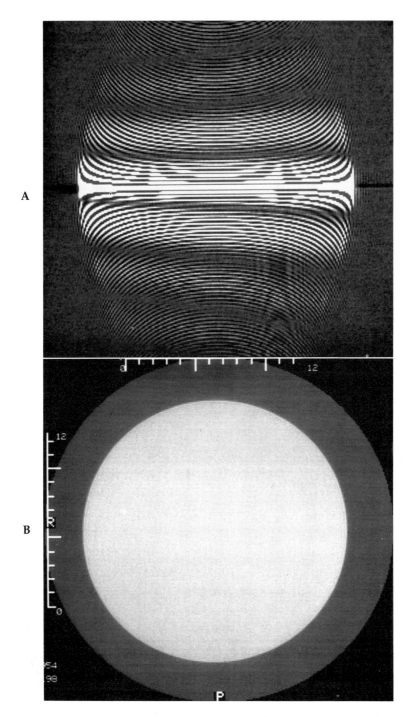

Fig. 4-15. **A,** Image processing is interrupted after the first FT of a spherical object revealing an intermediate image that is a crude frequency projection of the cross section of the object. **B,** After the second FT, the true image is reconstructed.

we can reconstruct the final image, which is homogeneous in signal and round in cross section (Fig. 4-15, *B*).

Q | **All this separate phase encoding and frequency encoding seems like such a bother. Why don't you just design gradients so that every pixel has a different frequency and frequency encode everything?**

This seems to be a great idea at first, but a few sketches will show you that it is impossible to construct a gradient field so that each pixel in a slice has a unique frequency. No matter how such a gradient is designed, there will always be two or more voxels with the same frequency; therefore, a scheme based on assigning a unique frequency to every point in a subject **simultaneously** is not tenable. It is possible, however, to oscillate the gradients so that *over time* each pixel is assigned a unique frequency. This strategy was used in the early days of MR imaging and formed the basis of *field-focused nuclear magnetic resonance* (FONAR) and other sensitive point techniques.

Reference

Morris PG. Nuclear magnetic resonance imaging in medicine and biology. Oxford: Clarendon, 1986, pp 78-90.

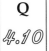

Q | **If each pixel is assigned a unique phase and frequency, why can't one use just a single phase-encoding step to determine the individual pixel values?**

Although frequency components can be uniquely decoded by Fourier transformation from a single echo, the individual phase shifts contributed by each pixel cannot. This lack of uniqueness of phase information can be easily illustrated by the following example.

Let pixel A emit an MR signal of the form $A(t) = \sin(\omega t + \phi_A)$, and let pixel B emit a signal $B(t) = \sin(\omega t + \phi_B)$. In an imaging experiment we measure an echo that contains the sum $A(t) + B(t)$. From the fundamental trigonometric identity $\sin X + \sin Y = 2 \sin \frac{1}{2}(X + Y) \cos \frac{1}{2}(X - Y)$, we find that

$$A(t) + B(t) = 2 \sin\{\omega t + \tfrac{1}{2}(\phi_A + \phi_B)\} \cos\{\tfrac{1}{2}(\phi_A - \phi_B)\}$$

This equation shows that the combination of the signals from A and B results in another sine wave of frequency ω. Although the base frequency (ω) remains unchanged when the signals from A and B combine, the phase shift of the resultant signal is $\frac{1}{2}(\phi_A + \phi_B)$. Because we record the summation signal $A(t) + B(t)$, not $A(t)$ and $B(t)$ individually, we are able to measure only the total resultant phase shift $\frac{1}{2}(\phi_A + \phi_B)$; we cannot know the individual phase contributions from A or B. Therefore, recording the MR signal after a single application of the phase-encoding gradient does not provide enough information to allow us to determine uniquely the pixel values corresponding to each phase location.

Q	**What is k-space?**
4.11	

K-space is perhaps the most confusing "catchword" to be thrust on the MR community in the last few years, but the confusion is unnecessary. K-space is a relatively simple concept we have been using all the time. We just did not call it k-space until recently.

Stated simply, k-space is an array of numbers whose FT is the MR image (Fig. 4-16). These numbers come from measuring the value of each MR signal at different times and plugging these values into the k-space array.

In routine 2DFT MR imaging, k-space is filled with data one row at a time (Fig. 4-17) by digitizing the MR signals obtained from the real (in phase) and imaginary (quadrature) channels. (Quadrature signal detection is discussed in Q 3.12, where I explain why we have two MR signals instead of one.) In this usual way of filling k-space by rows, the numbers placed in each cell correspond to the real and imaginary MR signal amplitudes at various times during the echo. The k-space values on the left side of each row are obtained early in the evolution of the echo, and those on the right side are obtained late. Note that in k-space, the center of the echo (and thus the largest values) occur near the middle of each row.

In 2DFT imaging, each row in k-space corresponds to the echo data obtained from a single application of the phase-encoding gradient (Fig. 4-18). By convention, rows near the center of the k-space grid are defined to correspond to low-order phase-encode steps, whereas those rows near the top and bottom correspond to higher-order phase encodings. Since echo amplitudes are larger at the low-order

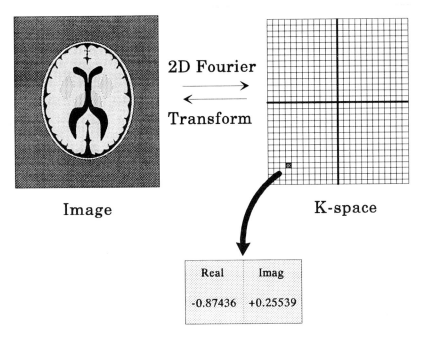

Fig. 4-16. K-space is simply a set of complex numbers (i.e., ones with real and imaginary components) whose 2DFT is the MR image.

phase-encode steps (there is less gradient-induced dephasing), the values of k-space are greater near the center of the grid.

Once all the phase-encode steps have been performed and all the echoes have been collected, digitized, and recorded, k-space is said to be *filled*. We can even display a picture of filled k-space, in which the brightness of each cell corresponds to the magnitude of the real or imaginary number assigned to that cell (Fig. 4-19, *A*). By performing a 2DFT of the k-space data, one obtains the corresponding MR image (Fig. 4-19, *D*).

It should be recognized that *individual cells in k-space do not correspond one to one with individual pixels in the MR image.* Each k-space cell contains information about every pixel in the image, and each pixel in the image is represented in every k-space cell. The k-space representation of the MR image is therefore more similar to the diffraction patterns generated by x-ray crystallography or holography than to the image on a photographic negative.

Finally, although there is no direct correspondence between the location of a cell in k-space and location of a pixel in the image, different parts of k-space do correspond topologically to spatial frequencies in the MR image. As illustrated in Fig. 4-20, data near the center of k-space correspond

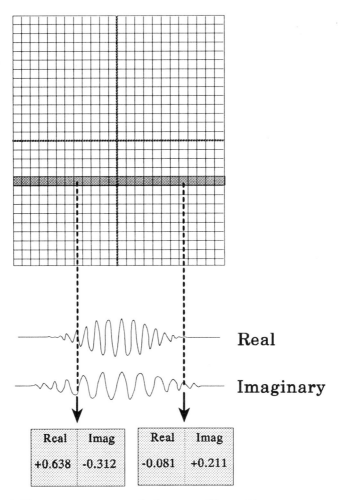

Fig. 4-17. In 2DFT spin warp imaging, the horizontal lines of k-space are acquired one by one. The real and imaginary numbers for each cell are the corresponding echo amplitudes in the real and imaginary data channels.

to low spatial frequencies (i.e., general shapes, contours), whereas data near the periphery contain information relating to high spatial frequencies (i.e., edges, details). This concept is demonstrated in Fig. 4-21, which shows an MR image constructed three ways: (1) using only the central data in k-space, (2) using only data from the periphery, and (3) using all the k-space data. When only the central data are used, a somewhat blurry image lacking spatial detail is generated. Conversely, when only peripheral data are used, an eerie image highlighting only edges and high-contrast details is apparent.

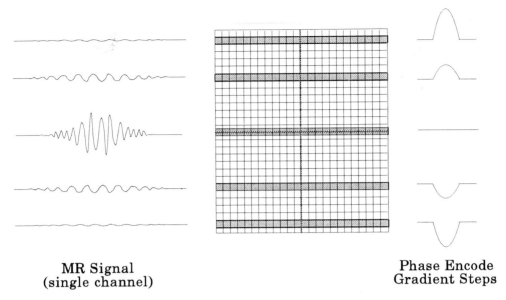

MR Signal
(single channel)

Phase Encode
Gradient Steps

Fig. 4-18. Global view of how echo data are used to fill k-space. By convention, low-order phase-encode steps fill the center of k-space, whereas high-order steps fill the periphery.

Q 4.12	How is the size of a pixel or voxel calculated from a given set of imaging parameters?

Everyone dealing with MR imaging should be able calculate pixel or voxel size on the basis of imaging parameters displayed on each image. Let us consider a voxel of height z, which is equivalent to the slice thickness, and in-plane dimensions x and y, which are determined by the field of view (FOV) and imaging matrix.

For both 2DFT and 3DFT, the in-plane pixel size is determined by parameters specified during frequency encoding and phase encoding of the MR signal. These scanning parameters include the FOV and imaging matrix ($N_x \times N_y$). The FOV is usually chosen to match the anatomical area of interest, with values ranging from as small as 12 cm (for a wrist) to 24 cm (for a head) up to 40 to 60 cm (for a body). On many scanners one is able to specify only a single FOV value, which is assumed to be a spherical diameter and to apply to all three dimensions (x, y, z). Some scanners, however, now allow the operator to select individual FOV values for each dimension (FOV_x, FOV_y, FOV_z). In other scanners, options such as "rectangular field of view" allow one to vary FOV_x and FOV_y over a more limited range.

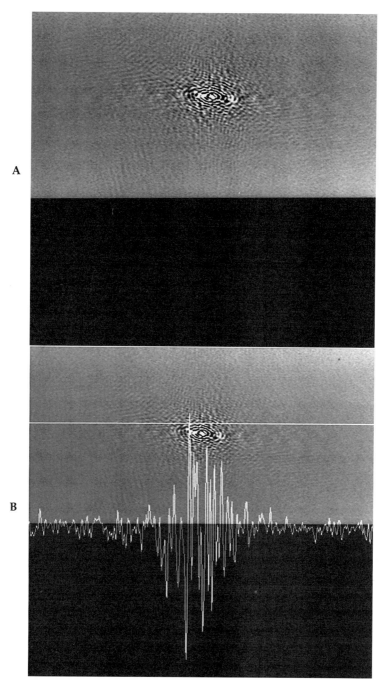

Fig. 4-19. A, Picture of k-space, with cell brightness corresponding to the magnitude of the number assigned to that cell. **B,** Data line near the center of k-space corresponds to values on a moderately high-amplitude echo.

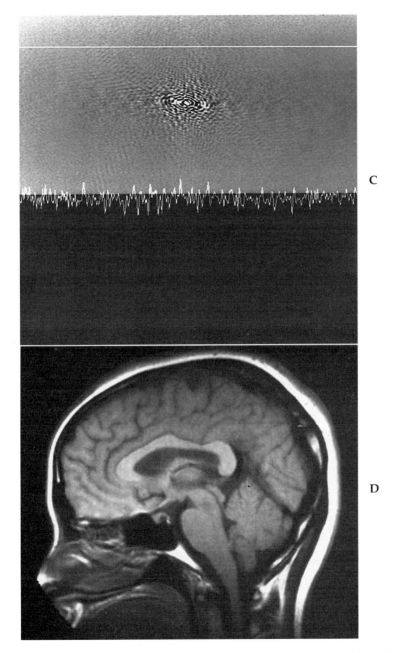

Fig. 4-19 (continued). **C,** Data line near the periphery of k-space corresponds to values of a low-amplitude echo obtained at a higher-order phase-encoding step. **D,** The MR image obtained by performing 2DFT on the k-space raw data.

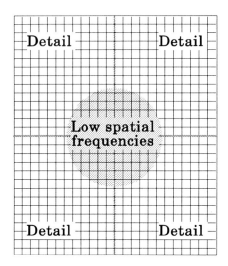

Fig. 4-20. The center of k-space contains low spatial frequencies (crude object shapes and contrasts). The periphery of k-space contains high spatial frequencies relating to image detail.

In addition to selecting the FOV, the operator must also select an in-plane imaging matrix size, denoted $(N_x \times N_y)$. In general, one of these values (N_x or N_y) represents the number of phase-encoding steps, and the other represents the number of frequency-encoding steps. Typical matrix sizes range from (128×256) to (512×512). The in-plane pixel dimensions for either 2DFT or 3DFT MR imaging are therefore

$$x = FOV_x/N_x \text{ and } y = FOV_y/N_y$$

How the height or depth of a voxel (z) is calculated depends on whether the image is acquired by 2DFT or 3DFT technique. For 2DFT imaging, z is the same as the slice thickness (THK) specified directly during scan prescription. For 3DFT imaging, one must know FOV_z, which is often called the slab thickness, as well as the number of phase-encoding steps in the z direction (N_z), sometimes identified as the number of 3D sections or partitions. The voxel depth z is therefore given by

$$z = THK \text{ (for 2DFT) or } z = FOV_z/N_z \text{ (for 3DFT)}$$

As a simple example, let us calculate the voxel size for a 3DFT spine study using a 19 cm FOV, a 192×256 imaging matrix, and a slab thickness of 16 cm with 64 partitions. The voxel dimensions are therefore

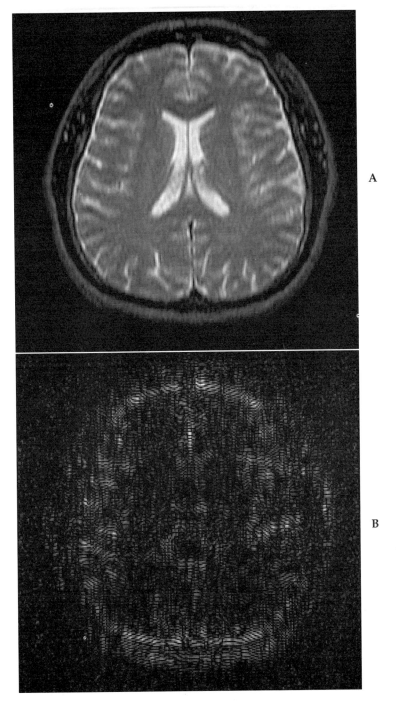

A

B

Fig. 4-21. **A,** Image reconstructed using data from the center 10% of k-space. **B,** Image reconstructed using data from the periphery of k-space showing edge detail.

Continued.

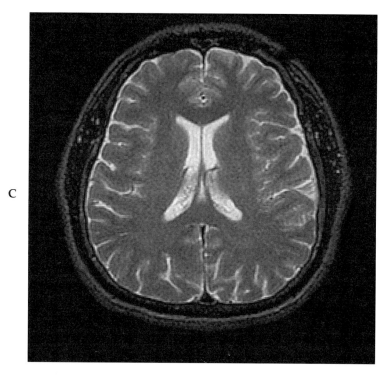

C

Fig. 4-21 (continued). **C,** Full image using all k-space data.

$$x = (19 \text{ cm})/192 = 0.10 \text{ cm} = 1.0 \text{ mm}$$

$$y = (19 \text{ cm})/256 = 0.07 \text{ cm} = 0.7 \text{ mm}$$

$$z = (16 \text{ cm})/64 = 0.25 \text{ cm} = 2.5 \text{ mm}$$

Q **How do you calculate the signal-to-noise ratio for an MR image?**

MR textbooks contain many complex equations defining the signal-to-noise ratio (SNR). These equations need not be memorized and can be quickly derived from the following simple expression:

$$\text{SNR} = K \cdot (\text{Voxel size}) \cdot \sqrt{\text{Measurements}} / \sqrt{\text{Bandwidth}}$$

Here K is a constant that includes the coil-filling factor, coil resistance, patient resistance, noise power spectrum, pulse sequence, and tissue parameters (T1, T2, spin density). *K* also depends on the operating frequency and therefore on magnetic field strength. Although some controversy still exists concerning the dependence of SNR on field strength, most physicists now agree that the dependence is approximately linear; *that is, $K \propto B_o$.*

It is easy to see why SNR should be proportional to voxel size: the larger the voxel, the larger the signal. Calculation of voxel size is discussed in Q 4.12, and the answer depends on whether the data were acquired as 2DFT or 3DFT:

$$\text{For 2DFT:} \quad \text{Voxel size} = \frac{FOV_x}{N_x} \cdot \frac{FOV_y}{N_y} \cdot THK$$

$$\text{For 3DFT:} \quad \text{Voxel size} = \frac{FOV_x}{N_x} \cdot \frac{FOV_y}{N_y} \cdot \frac{FOV_z}{N_z}$$

The term *measurements* represents the total number of signal components used in the Fourier reconstruction of the voxel. *"Measurements" is* not *synonymous with the number of excitations (NEX).* As with voxel size, the value of measurements depends on the mode of signal acquisition:

$$\text{For 2DFT: Measurements} = N_x \cdot N_y \cdot NEX$$

$$\text{For 3DFT: Measurements} = N_x \cdot N_y \cdot N_z \cdot NEX$$

One might wonder why SNR is proportional to the *square root* of measurements and not just to the number of measurements directly. The reason is that our equation computes the signal-to-noise *ratio,* not just the signal. Indeed, signal strength itself is proportional to the number of "measurements." Image noise, however, is assumed to be "white" (i.e., covering a wide range of frequencies) and uncorrelated from measurement to measurement. The noise, therefore, increases only with the square root of the number of measurements. We then have

$$\frac{\textbf{Signal}}{\textbf{Noise}} \propto \frac{\textbf{Measurements}}{\sqrt{\textbf{Measurements}}} = \sqrt{\textbf{Measurements}}$$

The receiver bandwidth (BW) represents the range of frequencies that span a pixel. Note that receiver BW is not the same as the RF transmitter BW discussed in Q 4.02. Receiver BW is defined as

$$\text{Bandwidth} = N_x / t_{samp}$$

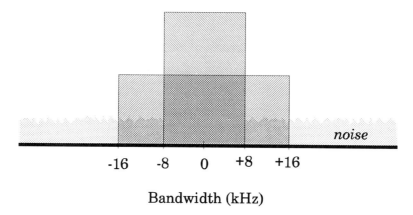

Bandwidth (kHz)

Fig. 4-22. Signal-to-noise ratio (SNR) as a function of signal bandwidth. Total signal energy is constant regardless of bandwidth, illustrated by the equal areas of the ±8 kHz and ±16 kHz spectra *(shaded rectangles)*. Image noise, assumed to be white, is uniformly distributed across all frequencies. Wider bandwidths encode more noise than narrow ones.

where t_{samp} = the sampling time. Because the noise is considered to be white (evenly distributed over all frequencies), when the BW is low (i.e., long sample times), less noise is encoded into the image. Conversely, large BWs span more frequencies and encode more noise (Fig. 4-22).

The true signal one is trying to detect, however, is generally independent of the receiver BW. That is, the signal is merely compressed or expanded to fit the specified BW. BW, then, principally affects the noise level, and the noise is statistical, again according to the square root of its size. This explains why $\sqrt{bandwidth}$ appears in the denominator of the SNR equation.

Substituting the values for 2DFT and 3DFT previously given in the simple SNR equation gives the complicated results found in many books:

$$\text{For 2DFT:}\quad \text{SNR} = K \cdot \frac{\text{FOV}_x}{N_x} \cdot \frac{\text{FOV}_y}{N_y} \cdot \text{THK} \cdot \frac{\sqrt{N_x}\,\sqrt{N_y}\,\sqrt{\text{NEX}}}{\sqrt{N_x}\,/\,\sqrt{t_{samp}}}$$

$$= K \cdot \frac{\text{FOV}_x}{N_x} \cdot \frac{\text{FOV}_y}{N_y} \cdot \text{THK} \cdot \sqrt{N_y} \cdot \sqrt{\text{NEX}} \cdot \sqrt{t_{samp}}$$

$$\text{For 3DFT:}\quad \text{SNR} = K \cdot \frac{\text{FOV}_x}{N_x} \cdot \frac{\text{FOV}_y}{N_y} \cdot \frac{\text{FOV}_z}{N_z} \cdot \frac{\sqrt{N_x}\,\sqrt{N_y}\,\sqrt{\sqrt{N_z}}\,\sqrt{\text{NEX}}}{\sqrt{N_x}\,/\,\sqrt{t_{samp}}}$$

$$= K \cdot \frac{\text{FOV}_x}{N_x} \cdot \frac{\text{FOV}_y}{N_y} \cdot \frac{\text{FOV}_z}{N_z} \cdot \sqrt{N_y} \cdot \sqrt{N_z} \cdot \sqrt{\text{NEX}} \cdot \sqrt{t_{samp}}$$

TABLE 4-1. Adjusting Imaging Parameters to Improve Signal-to-Noise Ratio (SNR)	
Change in Parameter	Disadvantage/Trade-off
Increasing voxel size ($\uparrow$ FOV, $\uparrow$ slice thickness, $\downarrow$ number of phase-encoding steps)	Decreases spatial resolution
Increasing number of signals averaged (NEX)	Increases imaging time disproportionately to gain in SNR (doubling NEX increases SNR by $\sqrt{2}$)
Using narrow bandwidth technique	Limits number of slices available for a given repetition time (TR); increases chemical shift artifacts; increases motion artifacts
Increasing interslice gap (reducing RF interference/cross-talk)	May miss lesions found only in the "gaps"
Using 3DFT instead of 2DFT acquisition (see Q 4.13)	Increases imaging time; increases motion artifacts
Reducing systematic noise (flow compensation, gating, antialiasing)	Various time and hardware limitations dependent on strategy selected

You should now better understand where all these factors and square roots in the SNR equations originated. A summary of the methods of improving the SNR and their relative disadvantages is presented in Table 4-1.

Q 4.14 **I've been told that SNR is much better for a 3DFT than a 2DFT sequence, but even after deriving all these equations, I still don't see why.**

Let us then look more closely at the SNR equations we have derived for 2DFT and 3DFT (see Q 4.13). Comparing these two sequences under conditions of equal slice thickness (i.e., set $THK = FOV_z/N_z$), we see that

$$SNR_{3DFT} = \sqrt{N_z} \cdot SNR_{2DFT}$$

so that SNR for the 3DFT technique is improved over the 2DFT technique by a factor of $\sqrt{N_z}$. In a 3DFT study with 64 partitions ($N_z = 64$), SNR gains by a factor of 8 compared with a 2DFT study. This seems too good to be true.

However, when we consider the imaging time for each sequence:

$$T_{2DFT} = TR \cdot N_y \cdot \text{NEX}$$

$$T_{3DFT} = TR \cdot N_y \cdot N_z \cdot \text{NEX}$$

where TR is repetition time, we easily see that

$$T_{3DFT} = N_z \cdot T_{2DFT}$$

Even though our 64-partition 3DFT study produced an increase in SNR by a factor of 8, imaging time has increased by a factor of 64! Clearly, 3DFT studies can be prohibitively long unless the TR is kept relatively short.

Q 4.15	What is meant by a "T1-weighted" or a "T2-weighted" image?

The terms *T1 weighted* and *T2 weighted* are among the most overused and least understood concepts in MR imaging. In the broadest sense, these terms are used to communicate to other radiologists and clinicians the type of MR pulse sequence employed to generate a series of images. "T1 weighted" usually refers to either a spin echo (SE) sequence with short TR/short TE or a spoiled gradient echo (GRE) technique; "T2 weighted" usually implies a long TR/long TE sequence; and "proton (spin) density weighted" usually means a long TR/short TE sequence. This shorthand notation of parameter weighting is thoroughly ingrained in the MR vocabulary, and I have no objection to its use in this form.

A fundamental misconception about a T1-weighted (or T2-weighted) image is that all tissue contrast in the image is dominated by T1 (or T2) effects. This literal interpretation of "T1 weighted" and "T2 weighted" is quite incorrect, since nearly all MR images display tissue contrasts that depend complexly on spin density, T1, and T2 simultaneously. Almost every MR image should properly be called "mixed" density. Furthermore, different tissues in different parts of an image may have completely different "weightings."

In 1988 I proposed a simple scheme for classifying the relative contributions of T1, T2, and spin density effects on image contrast for a given tissue and pulse sequence. This index system was based on computing fractional sensitivities for each MR parameter (i.e., % change in MR signal ÷ % change in T1, T2, or spin density.) Weighting indices for T1,

| | TABLE | 4-2. MR Parameter Weighting Indices for Brain at 0.35 T |

Pulse Sequence	T1-Weighting Index	T2-Weighting Index	Spin Density–Weighting Index
500/30	−28*	24	48
2000/60	−4	48	48
3000/30	−1	33	66
3000/120	0	66	34

*A negative index implies that lengthening T1 results in decreased signal intensity.

T2, and spin density could then be easily defined and scaled to be numbers between −1 and +1, and normalized so that their sum is 1.

When this mathematical analysis is performed, some rather surprising results are obtained (Table 4-2). For example, SE sequences such as 500/30, traditionally called "T1 weighted," actually produce images that depend more on changes in spin density than on T1; T2 effects also cannot be considered negligible. Proton (spin) density–weighted sequences, such as SE 3000/30, are accurate because they most reflect proton density; nevertheless, they have an appreciable contribution from T2 as well. Likewise, long TR/long TE sequences (e.g., 3000/120) have both T2 and spin density weighting, even though they are usually referred to as "T2 weighted." (See also Q 5.14, where I discuss the use and misuse of these terms with regard to GRE sequences.)

Reference

Elster AD. An index system for comparative parameter weighting in MR imaging. J Comput Assist Tomogr 12:130, 1988.

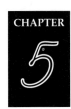
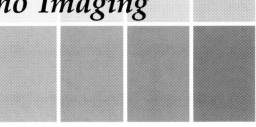

Gradient Echo Imaging

Gradient echo (GRE or GE) techniques are an essential component of the modern MR examination and are offered as standard software by every major vendor. They have proved useful in a wide variety of applications, including spinal imaging, cardiac imaging, MR angiography, three-dimensional imaging, echo planar imaging, and dynamic contrast techniques. Because of their great versatility, many GRE variations have been developed. In this chapter I attempt to answer some of the more frequently asked questions concerning GRE imaging.

Q	How does a gradient echo differ from a spin echo?
5.01	

A spin echo (SE) is produced by pairs of radiofrequency (RF) pulses, whereas a GRE is produced by a single RF pulse in conjunction with a gradient reversal. The formation of a GRE is illustrated schematically in Fig. 5-1. After the RF pulse, the first negative-going lobe of the gradient causes a phase dispersion of the precessing spins. When this gradient is reversed, the spins refocus and form a gradient (recalled) echo.

GRE imaging differs from SE imaging in several respects. First, because only one RF pulse has been applied, the echo can be recorded much more quickly in a GRE sequence. As a result, echo time (TE) is generally shorter for GRE sequences than for SE sequences. When GRE sequences are used with low–flip angle excitations (see Q 5.02), short values of repetition time (TR) may also be used. The combination of short TR and short TE values

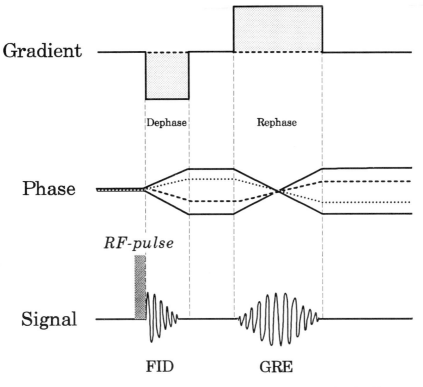

Fig. 5-1. Formation of a gradient echo (GRE). See Q 5.01 for details.

allows for very rapid signal acquisition. For this reason, GRE sequences form the basis for most rapid imaging and MR angiographic techniques.

A second important feature of GRE imaging is that *the gradient reversal refocuses only those spins that have been dephased by action of the gradient itself.* Specifically, phase shifts resulting from magnetic field inhomogeneities, static tissue susceptibility gradients, or chemical shifts are *not* canceled at the center of the GRE as they are in SE sequences. Image contrast is therefore dictated not by true T2 relaxation, but by these other factors that constitute T2* (see Q 2.11). GRE sequences are therefore more frequently troubled by susceptibility and chemical shift artifacts (see Q 6.01 and Q 6.06) and do not function well on scanners whose magnetic fields lack homogeneity.

Reference

Winkler ML, Ortendahl DA, Mills TC et al. Characteristics of partial flip angle and gradient reversal MR imaging. Radiology 166:17, 1988.

<table>
<tr><td>**Q**
5.02</td><td>**What is a partial flip angle pulse, and why would you want to use one?**</td></tr>
</table>

The term *partial flip angle* refers to the use of RF pulses that tip the longitudinal magnetization some fraction of 90° (e.g., 10°, 45°). Partial flip angle pulses are used widely in association with GRE techniques to minimize signal loss from saturation effects, as well as to provide a means for obtaining interesting new tissue contrasts.

Fig. 5-2 demonstrates schematically how a partial flip angle pulse creates an appreciable transverse magnetization while disturbing the longitudinal magnetization only slightly. From trigonometric identities, we see that when a magnetization vector **M** initially aligned with the z axis is flipped by angle α, the transverse and longitudinal components of magnetization after the flip are [M sin α] and [M cos α], respectively. For example, a 15° RF pulse acting on **M** creates an appreciable transverse component of size (sin 15°) × M, or 0.26 M, while reducing the longitudinal magnetization only 3% to (cos 15°) × M, or 0.97 M. Since longitudinal magnetization has been largely preserved, little saturation has occurred, and the next RF pulse will still have a large reservoir of magnetization from which to generate a signal. This advantage is particularly important when TR is short (i.e., < 100 msec). For short TR sequences, a significantly stronger MR signal may be obtained by using partial flip angle (rather than 90°) pulses.

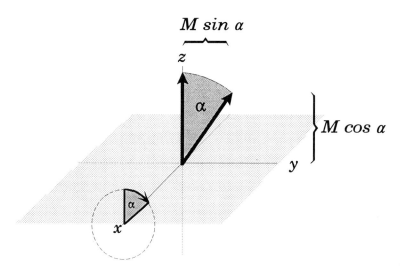

Fig. **5-2.** A partial flip angle (α) pulse can create an appreciable transverse magnetization [M sin α] while reducing the longitudinal magnetization [M cos α] only slightly. This results from the fundamental trigonometric property that cos α ≈ 1 for small values of α.

Reference

Mills TC, Ortendahl DA, Hylton NM et al. Partial flip angle MR imaging. Radiology 162:531, 1987.

Q | If a partial flip angle pulse tips *less* magnetization into the transverse plane than a 90° pulse, how can the signal be higher?

At first it seems paradoxical that reducing the flip angle (and thus the fraction of longitudinal magnetization deflected into the transverse plane) could ever generate a stronger signal than could be produced by using 90° pulses. Indeed, if only a single RF pulse were applied, then a 90° flip angle would always be optimal. However, an MR imaging sequence involves the application of *repetitive* RF pulses. These pulses, particularly if closely spaced, tend to reduce the size of the steady-state longitudinal magnetization (M_z), which is the magnetization flipped to create the MR signal. The overall signal therefore represents a "balancing act" between two factors: (1) the value of M_z and (2) the fraction of M_z tipped into the transverse plane by each pulse. Although 90° pulses tip the largest fraction of magnetization into the transverse plane, they also reduce the value of M_z, and overall MR signal is therefore not necessarily maximized. Conversely, partial flip angle pulses tip a smaller fraction of magnetization into the transverse plane but reduce M_z less. Overall, therefore, a series of partial flip angle pulses may generate a stronger signal than is generated by a series of 90° pulses.

Q | How do you know which flip angle to pick?

The flip angle maximizing the MR signal for a given tissue depends on the type of pulse sequence used and its imaging parameters. For sequences in which no transverse steady state is established, MR signal is maximized at the Ernst angle (α_E), which can be computed as

$$\cos \alpha_E = \exp(-TR/T1)$$

Note that this equation predicts that the optimal flip angle will be 90° only when TR >> T1.

As an example, let us calculate the optimal flip angle for such a sequence in the brain, where the average T1 = 800 msec. When TR = 3000 msec, the Ernst angle is computed to be 89°. In this situation, conventional 90° pulses are nearly optimal. When TR = 100 msec, however, a different result is obtained; the optimal angle is calculated to be only 28°.

The actual boost in signal obtained by using optimized flip angles is surprisingly large. For example, consider a spoiled-GRE sequence (Q 5.09) whose theoretical signal intensity is given by

$$Signal \propto M_o \frac{1 - \exp(-TR/T1)}{1 - \exp(-TR/T1)\, \cos\alpha} \sin\alpha$$

Let us compute the expected signal from brain for two flip angles, 15° and 90°, for such a sequence with TR = 30 msec (here, 15° is close to the Ernst angle). The calculated signal at 15° is 0.132 M_o, but the signal at 90° is only 0.009 M_o. In this example we see that with an appropriate choice of flip angle, the MR signal can be boosted by a factor of 14.7 over that obtainable by using 90° pulses.

Reference

Ernst RR, Anderson WA. Application of Fourier transform spectroscopy to magnetic resonance. Rev Sci Instrum 37:93, 1966. (This article contains in-depth physics, but is a classic.)

| Q 5.05 | **Partial flip angles seem to be used only in GRE imaging. Why can't you use them with spin echo techniques as well?** |

You *can* use partial flip angles in SE imaging, as long as certain precautions are observed.

In general, performing an SE sequence of the form α°-180°-echo creates several problems with the maintenance of longitudinal magnetization that are not a concern in GRE imaging. The source of this problem in SE imaging stems from the use of 180° pulses. These 180° pulses play a vital role in routine SE imaging, flipping over the transverse magnetization within its plane and thereby compensating for the effect of static field inhomogeneities. In routine SE imaging, however, the 180° pulses occur soon after the 90° pulses have deflected *all* the longitudinal magnetization into the transverse plane. This would not be the case, however, if the first pulse were α° (instead of 90°).

If a partial flip angle pulse were employed, the 180° pulse would do much more than merely compensate for field inhomogeneities. Not only would spins be flipped over in the transverse plane by this pulse, but so would the residual longitudinal magnetization (which could be considerable, since the α° pulse may have reduced it by only a small fraction). Thus the 180° pulse would invert the longitudinal magnetization, destroying the individual beneficial aspects of *both* partial flip angle and SE imaging.

Nevertheless, it is possible to work around this limitation. If one adds a 180° pulse at the end of the sequence, the longitudinal magnetization can be returned to its steady-state alignment along the +z axis with relatively little penalty incurred from the first 180° pulse. The simplest way to do this is merely to require the sequence to have an even number of echoes (i.e., to be of the form α° − 180° − echo − 180° − echo). Alternatively, if only a single echo is desired, one may use a *large* flip angle SE technique of the form α°-180°-echo, where α > 90°. Both techniques have been used with limited success and are available as commercial options on some scanners (e.g., Picker's THRIFT).

References

Elster AD, Provost TJ. Large-tip-angle spin echo imaging: theory and applications. Invest Radiol 1993 (in press).

Mitchell DG, Vinitski S, Burk DL Jr et al. Variable-flip-angle spin-echo MR imaging of the pelvis: more versatile T2-weighted images. Radiology 171:525, 1989.

Q 5.06	What's the difference between a gradient echo, a gradient-recalled echo, and a field echo?

They are all the same.

Q 5.07	It seems as if every manufacturer has adopted a different name for their GRE pulse sequences. Can you sort these out for me?

Unfortunately, no uniform system of nomenclature for GRE sequences has been adopted by MR manufacturers. To date, more than 40 different names, abbreviations, and acronyms have been devised by different vendors to

TABLE 5-1. Classification and Nomenclature of Gradient Echo (GRE) Sequences

Generic Name	Description	GE Name	Siemens Name
Spoiled GRE	Coherence of transverse magnetization is spoiled/disrupted.	SPGR "Spoiled GRASS"	FLASH "Fast Low-Angle Shot"
Steady-state GRE with free induction decay (FID) sampling	Transverse coherence is preserved; FID signal is sampled.	GRASS "Gradient-Recalled Acquisition in the Steady State"	FISP "Fast Imaging with Steady-State Precession"
Steady-state GRE with spin echo (SE) sampling	Transverse coherence is preserved; SE signal is sampled.	SSFP "Steady-State Free Precession"	PSIF "Mirrored FISP"
Magnetization-prepared GRE	Rapid GRE sequence with preparatory pulses.	Fast SPGR prepared	Turbo-FLASH MP-RAGE (3D) "Magnetization-Prepared Rapid Gradient Echo"

differentiate and market their products. To help straighten out all these confusing acronyms, I tabulated the ones in common use in 1993 and proposed a vendor-independent nomenclature. The complete list for 11 brands of scanners can be found in this reference, but most students should at least be familiar with the names used by the two largest manufacturers of MR scanners, GE Medical Systems and Siemens. These terms are summarized in Table 5-1. Other less common GRE acronyms can be found in the Appendix and in the table reference.

Reference

Elster AD. Gradient echo imaging: techniques and acronyms. Radiology 186:1, 1993.

 Q 5.08

What is meant by spoiling, and how is it accomplished?

Spoiling refers to the purposeful disruption of transverse coherences, which may persist from cycle to cycle in a GRE sequence when the TR is very short (i.e., TR < 50 to 100 msec). Spoiling ensures that immediately before each RF pulse, the steady-state magnetization has no transverse components. In other words, spoiling ensures that the steady-state magnetization points totally in the z direction before it is acted on by the next RF pulse.

Spoiled-GRE pulse sequences are offered by all MR manufacturers and marketed under familiar names such as FLASH, SPGR, RF-FAST, and T1-FAST. Although the final images produced by these sequences may appear nearly identical, several quite different spoiling methods are used by different manufacturers.

Gradient spoiling is performed by turning on the slice-select gradient an additional time, with variable amplitude at the end of each cycle immediately before the next RF pulse. The amplitude of this spoiler gradient is varied linearly or semirandomly from view to view. The Siemens' FLASH technique is the prototype gradient-spoiled sequence.

RF spoiling is accomplished by semirandomly changing the phase of the RF carrier from view to view. In theory, RF spoiling is superior to gradient spoiling because it does not generate eddy currents and is spatially invariant. GE Medical Systems' SPGR sequence is the prototype RF-spoiled sequence.

Reference

Elster AD. Gradient echo imaging: techniques and acronyms. Radiology 186:1, 1993.

Q 5.09

When would you want to use a spoiled-GRE technique? How do you pick the parameters?

Because the spoiled-GRE technique is specifically designed to disrupt transverse (T2) coherences, its major benefit and use are in producing proton density–weighted and T1–weighted images. When operated with short TR values (~50 msec) in a single-slice (two-dimensional Fourier transform, 2DFT) mode, the spoiled-GRE technique may be useful for imaging the liver or chest, since each image can be acquired during a few seconds of breath holding. The 2DFT mode may also be useful for dynamic enhancement studies of the brain, liver, or kidneys when gadolinium is administered by bolus infusion. Multislice (three-dimensional Fourier transform, 3DFT) spoiled-GRE sequences are also becoming popular and are now widely used in a variety of cranial and spinal applications.

TABLE	5-2. How to Manipulate Image Contrast in Spoiled-GRE Sequences	
Parameter	Action of Imaging Parameter	Image Contrast Created
Repetition time (TR)	Determines optimal flip angle (Ernst angle), which becomes smaller as TR is decreased	Little independent effect as long as α is properly scaled
Echo time (TE)	Determines degree of T2* weighting	Long TE → T2* weighting
Flip angle (α)	Controls relative spin density (ρ) and T1 weighting	Large α → T1 weighted Small α → ρ weighted

In selecting parameters appropriate for a given application, three points should be considered. First, to minimize T2 effects and thus maximize proton density weighting and T1 weighting, sequence TE should be as short as possible, preferably less than 10 to 15 msec. Second, reasonably wide latitude is permitted in the choice of TR, with values of 25 to 80 msec usually producing good-quality images. The lowest allowable TR in this range should generally be selected to minimize scan time. As a rule, better-quality images are obtained from a spoiled-GRE sequence using a very short TR and two excitations than using a TR twice as long with only one excitation, although both methods take the same amount of time. Third, flip angle is usually selected to maximize the spoiled-GRE signal once a TR and tissue of interest are selected. Flip angle (α) can be estimated by the classical Ernst angle equation (see Q 5.04), namely, $\cos \alpha_E = \exp(-TR/T1)$. For routine brain and spinal imaging, flip angles of 20° to 45° in conjunction with short TR values (30 to 50 msec) empirically provide the best-quality images. All other parameters being equal, low flip angles accentuate proton density weighting, whereas large flip angles accentuate T1 effects. As α approaches 90°, signal behavior of the spoiled-GRE sequence becomes similar to that of conventional SE imaging.

Spoiled-GRE techniques may also be used to produce T2*-weighted images, although this type of contrast is often better achieved using steady-state coherent GRE sequences. T2* effects can be maximized in the spoiled-GRE sequence by using long TR, long TE, and small-to-intermediate values of α. A summary of these contrast effects for various spoiled-GRE parameters is displayed in Table 5-2. Typical spoiled-GRE protocols in common use and the reasons for selecting different parameters are presented in Table 5-3.

TABLE 5-3. Typical Spoiled-GRE Protocols

Type of Image Contrast Desired	Parameter Selection	Reason
T1 weighting	Short TR (20-80 msec) Short TE (5-10 msec) Intermediate α (30°-50°) (This combination of parameters is the most widely used.)	T1 contrast would theoretically be better for α = 60°-90°, but signal would be weak because this is far from the Ernst angle. α = 30°-50° is a compromise for good signal and T1 contrast at short TR values.
	"Long" TR (100-400 msec) Short TE (5-10 msec) Large α (60°-90°)	Behaves as a SE sequence as α approaches 90°. "Long" TR is really "short" in SE terms. Short TE minimizes T2* effects.
Proton density weighting	"Long" TR (100-400 msec) Short TE (5-10 msec) Small α (5°-20°)	"Long" TR and small α minimize T1 weighting. Short TE minimizes T2* effects.
T2* weighting	"Very long" TR (200-500 msec) "Long" TE (20-50 msec) Small α (5°-20°)	"Very long" TR and small α minimize T1 effects. "Long" TE maximizes T2* contrast. Longer TEs are not practical because of susceptibility-related signal losses.

Reference

Haacke EM, Wielopolski PA, Tkach JA. A comprehensive technical review of short TR, fast, magnetic resonance imaging. Rev Magn Reson Med 3:53, 1991. (A whole issue in which many of the detailed technical features of steady-state imaging are explained.)

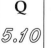

Q 5.10   **Can I use a spoiled-GRE sequence in place of conventional short TR/TE spin echo sequences?**

The answer to this question is not known, but the reader should be aware of the advantages and disadvantages of using spoiled-GRE rather than usual T1-weighted SE sequences.

Advantages. 3DFT spoiled-GRE sequences have the advantage of volumetric, thin-slice imaging, with no interslice gaps or cross-talk. Multiplanar reformatting is also possible. Flow artifacts are reduced. Excellent gray matter–white matter contrast may be achieved by this technique. Imaging time may be reduced.

Disadvantages. Image contrast with spoiled-GRE sequences may not be *exactly* the same as with conventional SE images. Some tissues occasionally differ significantly in signal intensity between spoiled-GRE and SE imaging. Susceptibility artifacts may hinder diagnosis in some areas, such as the skull base. Gadolinium enhancement in some tumors and infarctions may not be as apparent on the spoiled-GRE images as on SE ones.

Q 5.11	What is meant by a steady-state free precession?

A steady-state free precession may occur whenever a long series of closely spaced RF pulses is applied to a sample (Fig. 5-3). In this scenario, free induction decay (FID) signals occur after each RF pulse, and SEs are produced by successive pairs of RF pulses. Each set of three or more RF pulses in turn produces stimulated echoes (STEs), which coincide with the SEs when the RF pulses are evenly spaced and no gradients are applied for imaging. Moreover, if the RF pulses are applied sufficiently rapidly (i.e., TR << T2), the tails of the FIDs and SEs merge so that a continuous signal

STEADY-STATE FREE PRECESSION

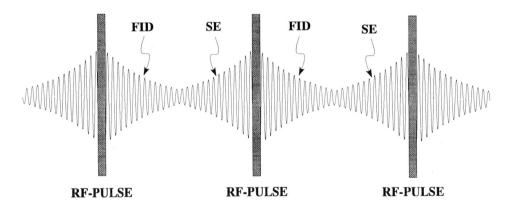

Fig. 5-3. Steady-state free precession signal is composed of superimposed free induction decay signals (FIDs), spin echoes (SEs), and stimulated echoes (STEs) summing together from multiple previous cycles.

of varying amplitude is produced, and a *steady-state free precession* becomes established.

The MR signal never completely fading out between RF pulses is equivalent to saying the transverse components of magnetization never fully dephase. This unique situation can occur only under special conditions: (1) TR must be significantly shorter than T2, or natural decay processes will destroy the transverse coherence; (2) phase shifts caused by imaging gradients must remain constant from cycle to cycle; (3) field inhomogeneities must be static; and (4) the spins must be stationary or motion compensated.

When a steady-state free precession becomes established, therefore, the magnetization that exists immediately before each RF pulse does not point along the +z axis as shown in the simplified representation of Fig. 5-2. Instead, this magnetization is obliquely oriented and possesses a nonzero transverse component in the *xy* plane (Fig. 5-4). The angle (β) at which this transverse magnetization lies in the *xy* plane is called the *resonant offset angle, phase angle,* or *precession angle.* Fig. 5-5 demonstrates how strongly the action of an RF pulse depends on the resonant offset.

Numerous artifacts and problems may arise in steady-state GRE imaging because of clustering and nonuniformity of resonant offset angles from pixel to pixel across the image. If a position-dependent distribution of resonant offset angles exists across a slice at the end of a cycle, the next RF pulse will have an effect on this signal that is also position dependent. As a result, bands of varying signal intensity (sometimes called "FLASH bands") may appear and significantly degrade the MR image (Fig. 5-6).

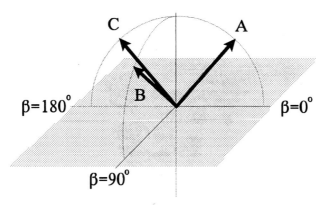

Fig. 5-4. Resonant offset (precession) angle, β. Spins *A, B,* and *C* have the same polar angle but different resonant offsets.

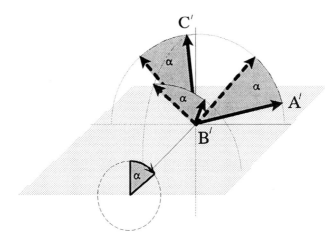

Fig. 5-5. Action of an α° RF pulse on a spin depends on both its initial polar angle and its resonant offset (β). A′, B′, and C′ represent the final positions of spins *A*, *B*, and *C* after an α° RF pulse.

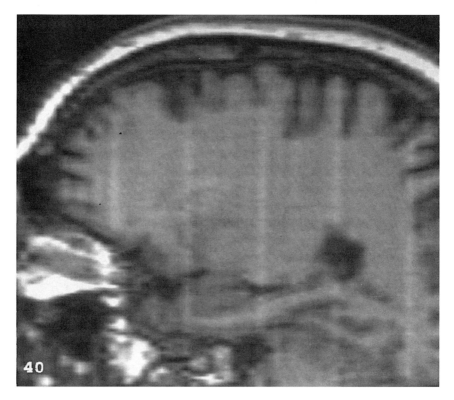

Fig. 5-6. "FLASH bands" are artifacts caused by position-dependent clustering of resonant offset angles from cycle to cycle in a GRE sequence.

References

Carr HY. Steady-state free precession in nuclear magnetic resonance. Phys Rev 112:1673, 1958. (Another paper with in-depth mathematics and physics, but serious MR students should have it in their libraries.)

Elster AD. Gradient echo imaging: techniques and acronyms. Radiology 186:1, 1993.

Q 5.12	How do you get rid of these "FLASH bands" and control resonant offset effects?

Steady-state GRE sequences control resonant offset effects and maintain steady-state coherence in two principal ways: (1) through *resonant offset averaging* in the read and slice-select directions and (2) through the application of *rewinder gradients* on the phase-encode axis. These techniques are illustrated schematically in Fig. 5-7.

Resonant offset averaging is accomplished by prolonging the duration of the read (and sometimes slice-select) gradient after echo collection.

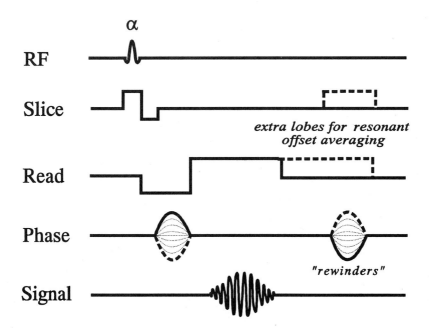

Fig. 5-7. Methods to eliminate FLASH bands and control resonant offset artifacts: (1) extra lobes for resonant offset averaging and (2) rewinder gradients.

These gradients are left on long enough to ensure that a full range of resonant offset angles (0° to 360°) exists across each voxel at the end of each cycle. This uniform redistribution of spin phase angles before the next RF pulse means the contribution to the steady-state magnetization is smoothed or averaged over all values of β. Accordingly, position-dependent changes in signal intensity and phase are minimized.

Rewinder gradients are a second set of phase-encoding steps applied with reverse polarity at the end of every cycle. The purpose of these rewinders is to ensure stability of the phase of the MR signal in each repetition interval and to aid in the development of coherent transverse magnetization. Without rewinders, resonant offset angles would vary from cycle to cycle because the phase-encode step changes. Phase-encoded information in one cycle could therefore "spill over" into the next cycle, generating unwanted STEs and FLASH bands in the image.

Reference

Elster AD. Gradient echo imaging: techniques and acronyms. Radiology 186:1, 1993.

Q 5.13	What is the difference between *coherent* and *incoherent* steady-state sequences?

As originally defined by Carr and Hahn, the term *steady-state free precession* should be applied to conditions in which coherence of transverse spins is maintained. Strictly speaking, therefore, a spoiled-GRE sequence such as FLASH should not be considered a steady-state free precession sequence, since the transverse coherences are destroyed. However, primarily because of the writings of Mark Haacke, a prominent GRE researcher, spoiled-GRE sequences are sometimes referred to as *steady-state incoherent*, whereas "true" steady-state free precession sequences are classified as *steady-state coherent*. The terms *coherent* and *incoherent* refer to the state of the transverse magnetization immediately before each RF pulse. Steady-state coherent techniques can be further subdivided into those that sample principally the FID component of the steady-state free precession signal and those that sample the SE/STE contributions. We have called those sequences that sample the FID components SS-GRE-FID and those that sample the SE/STE components SS-GRE-SE in our vendor-independent nomenclature.

Reference

Haacke EM, Tkach JA. Fast MR imaging: techniques and applications. AJR 155:951, 1990.

| Q 5.14 | How do you select imaging parameters for GRASS/FISP sequences? |

Steady-state sequences such as GRASS and FISP (see Table 5-1), which sample the FID signal, are among the most widely used of all GRE techniques. Because both longitudinal and transverse steady-state components of magnetization exist at the end of each cycle, repetitive RF pulses create a "mixing" or exchange of magnetization among the components (Fig. 5-8). The overall MR signal is therefore a summation of effects that

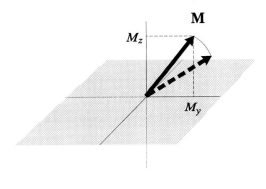

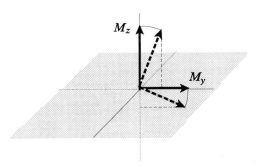

Fig. 5-8. Steady-state free precession sequence. If the magnetization vector **(M)** has nonzero transverse components at the end of a cycle, the next RF pulse induces a mixing of its transverse and longitudinal components.

take place over many cycles. Because of this complexity, it is impossible to explain easily (except in a few limiting cases) why different tissues appear the way they do over a wide range of imaging parameters. Unlike the relatively simple equations for calculating signal intensity for SE or spoiled-GRE sequences, the signal intensity equations derived for GRASS/FISP are extremely complex, incorporating linear and exponential combinations of terms that include T1, T2, T2*, T2/T1, and flip angle (α), as well as integrals whose values depend on RF-phase relationships and the net effect of imaging gradients. Despite this complexity, a few basic statements concerning image contrast in these sequences are possible.

GRASS/FISP contrast is perhaps the easiest to understand when the assumptions of a coherent transverse steady state break down (see Q 5.11). For example, when TR is much longer than T2 (e.g., TR > 200 msec for most tissues), natural T2 decay processes intrinsically spoil the sequence and convert it to spoiled-GRE behavior. Physiological motion may also contribute to this intrinsic spoiling of the GRASS/FISP sequence. Thus, flowing cerebrospinal fluid (CSF) and blood may exhibit spoiled contrast behavior, even though stationary tissue is in a steady-state free precession.

For shorter values of TR, both a longitudinal and a transverse steady state become established, and image contrast is dictated principally by α. As I subsequently demonstrate, low flip angles ($\alpha < 20°$) produce spin density–weighted images, whereas larger flip angles ($\alpha > 45°$) result in contrast that is sensitive to the ratio T2/T1.

As explained in Q 5.02, a low–flip angle pulse creates an appreciable transverse magnetization while disturbing the longitudinal magnetization only slightly. When α is small, therefore, most of the steady-state magnetization remains in the longitudinal direction, a phenomenon dependent primarily on the trigonometric fact that cos $\alpha \approx 1$ for small α (and thus essentially independent of tissue T1 or T2). Stated another way, the longitudinal magnetization does not change much after a small α pulse, regardless of the T1 or T2 value. For low flip angles, therefore, image contrast depends primarily on the equilibrium magnetization, which reflects the total number of spins in the sample. Thus, low flip angles ($\alpha < 20°$) produce spin density–weighted images.

When α is large, however, considerable interchange between the longitudinal and transverse magnetization components occurs with each pulse. The net signal then depends strongly on both T1 and T2, or more explicitly, on the *ratio* T2/T1. For most solid tissues, T1 is approximately 5 to 10 times longer than T2, but for fluids, T2 and T1 are nearly equal. As α increases, therefore, the signal from CSF and other fluids significantly increases because of this T2/T1 behavior.

The TE in a GRE sequence adjusts sensitivity to T2* effects. As discussed in Q 2.12, T2* represents the effective or observed T2, which is a manifestation of "true" tissue T2, as well as field inhomogeneities and susceptibility changes. In general, T2* is much shorter than T2; its range is usually 5 to 15 msec for most tissues in a 1.5 T scanner. "Short" TE therefore means values less than 15 msec. "Long" TE usually is satisfied for values of 30 to 60 msec.

A summary of these image contrast manipulations appears in Table 5-4, and typical GRASS/FISP protocols with the reasons for the various choices of parameters are listed in Table 5-5. The reader should realize that terms such as *T1 weighting* and *T2* weighting* are not strictly defined and that in a single image, many different tissue contrasts may be present simultaneously. For example, some parts of a GRASS/FISP image may exhibit T1 contrast, whereas other parts show T2/T1 contrast and spin density weighting. Furthermore, the signal from water/CSF cannot be used as a simple and reliable guide to the type of weighting as it can in SE imaging. Water may be equally bright on spin density–, T2*-, and T2/T1-weighted steady-state GRE images.

TABLE 5-4. How to Manipulate Contrast in GRASS/FISP Sequences

Parameter	Action of Imaging Parameter	Image Contrast Created
Repetition time (TR)	Determines whether a steady-state free precession (SSFP) is permitted to exist.	TR long→steady state is spoiled. Use Table 5-2 to predict effects of α. TR short→steady state *may* exist, provided it is not spoiled by motion or gradients (nonsequential multislice mode).
Echo time (TE)	Controls sensitivity to T2* effects.	Long TE→T2* weighting.
Flip angle (α)	Controls degree of mixing of transverse and longitudinal steady-state components.	Small α→spin density (ρ) weighting. Large α →T2/T1 weighting.

TABLE	5-5. Typical GRASS/FISP Protocols	

Type of Image Contrast Desired	Parameter Selection	Reason
T1 weighting	"Long" TR (200-400 msec) Short TE (5-15 msec) Large α (45°-90°)	"Long" TR means T2 coherences cannot be maintained, and sequence behaves as spoiled GRE. Short TE minimizes T2* effects. Large α accentuates T1 contrast when TR is long.
Proton density weighting	"Long" TR (200-400 msec) Short TE (5-15 msec) Small α (5°-20°)	"Long" TR and short TE minimize T2 and T2* effects. Small α reduces T1 sensitivity and makes sequence primarily dependent on spin density.
T2* weighting	"Long" TR (100-400 msec) "Long" TE (25-60 msec) Small α (5°-20°)	As for proton density parameters, but longer TE accentuates T2* contribution.
T2/T1 weighting	Short TR (20-50 msec) Short TE (5-15 msec) Large α (40°-90°)	As α increases, signal becomes more dependent on T2/T1. Signal from liquids is accentuated because T2/T1 is much larger in liquids than in solids.

Reference

Haacke EM, Frahm J. A guide to understanding key aspects of fast gradient-echo imaging. JMRI 1:621, 1991.

Q 5.15 Why is there a difference in contrast behavior between GRASS/FISP sequences obtained in the sequential (single-slice) mode and those obtained in the interleaved (slice-multiplexed) mode? How about between 2DFT and 3DFT acquisitions?

When very short TR values are employed, it is usually possible to obtain only a single GRASS/FISP slice at a time. To cover a large area, therefore, a series of individual GRASS/FISP images must be acquired; this technique is called *sequential multislice acquisition.*

If longer TR values are employed, it is possible to use slice multiplexing (as in conventional SE imaging) to acquire several slices simultaneously within a TR interval. This method is known as *slice-interleaved* or *slice-multiplexed acquisition*.

In the sequential multislice mode, each slice is acquired independently and has the signal characteristics shown in Tables 5-4 and 5-5. Furthermore, each slice can be considered an "entry slice" with respect to flow effects. Therefore, inflow enhancement effects of blood or CSF are maximal when this mode of acquisition is used.

In the slice-multiplexed mode, however, a significantly different behavior can be expected. Because multiple slices must be selected during each TR interval, a slice-select gradient must be turned on for each slice imaged. These slice-select gradients spoil transverse coherences and convert the GRASS/FISP sequence to display spoiled-GRE contrast. Also in this mode, because only the end slices are true "entry slices," inflow enhancement effects are less pronounced.

Finally, somewhat different contrast behavior may be seen when a GRASS/FISP sequence is operated in the 2DFT and 3DFT modes. As far as flow effects are concerned, the interior slices of a 3DFT acquisition are even less inclined to exhibit inflow enhancement than those of the 2DFT-multiplexed sequence. Overall image contrast may also vary among different parts of the 3DFT volume; this effect is caused by the difficulty in obtaining a uniform RF flip angle throughout the volume. As the flip angle varies, so does image contrast.

Reference

Wehrli F. Fast scan magnetic resonance imaging. New York: Raven, 1989, p 41.

Q	**What's the difference between FISP and PSIF?**
5.16	

PSIF is Siemens' acronym for a steady-state GRE sequence that samples the SE/STE components of the free precession signal rather than the FID (see Table 5-1). PSIF is a reversal of the letters in the acronym FISP and is appropriate because the pulse-timing diagrams for FISP and PSIF are mirror images of each other. GE Medical Systems calls its version of this sequence SSFP. This initialing is somewhat misleading, however, since *both* FISP and PSIF are steady-state free precession sequences.

Image contrast in the PSIF sequence is even more difficult to explain on an intuitive level, since the echo recorded is actually brought down into the transverse plane by an RF pulse in the preceding cycle. The effective TE is thus TR + TE, since an entire additional cycle (of length TR) has passed before echo collection. This relatively large evolutionary period before echo collection allows for natural transverse decay of the magnetization to occur. Images from PSIF sequences thus appear to have a prominent T2 weighting regardless of the other parameters chosen. Because T2 contrast is apparently "enhanced" by this technique, the acronym "contrast-enhanced FAST" or "CE-FAST" was the original name given to this sequence; it has been retained by Picker in the name of the company's commercial version.

Reference

Gyngell ML. The application of steady-state free precession in rapid 2DFT NMR imaging: FAST and CE-FAST sequences. Magn Reson Imaging 6:415, 1988.

Q 5.17 | What's the difference between FLASH and Turbo-FLASH?

Turbo-FLASH is essentially a FLASH sequence run more rapidly than usual, with additional interesting consequences (see Table 5-1). When a GRE sequence is run with *extremely* short TR values (i.e., TR < T2*), neither a longitudinal nor a transverse steady state has enough time to become fully established during the course of an imaging experiment. Since the T2*s of most tissues in 1.5 T scanners are less than 20 msec, Turbo-FLASH sequences are typically run with TR values of 10 msec or less. Because image acquisition has not taken place under steady-state conditions, nonuniform weighting of data occurs along the phase-encoded axis, with subsequent loss of image resolution. Furthermore, because the TR values are so short, small flip angles must be used to minimize saturation and to preserve signal-to-noise ratio. As a result, image contrast for the simple Turbo-FLASH sequence is dominated by spin density effects and is therefore relatively poor. Nevertheless, simple Turbo-FLASH-like sequences can be useful in dynamic gadolinium-enhanced studies to quantitate contrast uptake.

Despite this intrinsically poor contrast of Turbo-FLASH, interesting contrast behavior may be restored by applying a preparatory pulse (or pulses) in the interval before beginning data collection. When modified in this fashion, these sequences are called *magnetization-prepared* rapid GRE techniques. Siemens calls them MP-RAGE, and GE Medical Systems refers to them as SPGR prepared.

Reference

Chien D, Edelman RR. Ultrafast imaging using gradient echoes. Magn Reson Q 1:31, 1991.

Q	**What types of preparatory pulses are available?**
5.18	

The simplest preparatory pulse is simply a nonselective or "hard" 180° pulse that inverts the tissue magnetization across the sample. After an inversion time delay (TI), a 2DFT or 3DFT Turbo-GRE sequence is performed. Image contrast is determined by the effective TI for this sequence, which is the time interval between the 180° pulse and the central phase-encoding step. Because the equilibrium magnetization (and thus T1 contrast) may be changing during this sequence, it is potentially important to have control over the ordering of the phase-encode steps. Final image contrast depends on the precise order in which the phase-encode lines have been sampled. Additionally, if rapid T1 relaxation occurs during data acquisition, segmentation of the total sequence into several steps, including waiting periods, may be necessary.

By changing the preparatory period to a 90°/180°/−90° set of pulses, T2 contrast can be obtained. This is the so-called driven-equilibrium (DE) version of the sequence. Other proposed preparatory period variations include schemes to produce STEs, diffusion weighting, and magnetization transfer sensitivity. Expect many advances in this major growth area within the next few years.

Reference

Mugler JP III, Brookeman JR. Three-dimensional magnetization-prepared rapid gradient-echo imaging. Magn Reson Med 15:152, 1990.

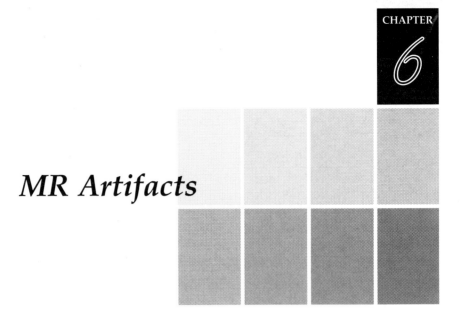

MR Artifacts

The recognition and correction of artifacts is an important aspect of clinical MR imaging. In this chapter I answer questions concerning some common MR artifacts encountered daily in MR imaging and explain both why they occur and what can be done to overcome them.

| Q 6.01 | What is a chemical shift artifact? |

As discussed in Q 2.16 to Q 2.18, the term *chemical shift* refers to the change in a hydrogen proton's local magnetic field (and thus resonant frequency) as a function of the molecular environment in which it resides. For example, the protons of fatty triglycerides are chemically shielded by their electron clouds and therefore resonate at slightly lower frequencies than do water protons in the same tissue. This shift in resonant frequency has been measured to be approximately 3.5 parts per million (ppm), or a difference of about 225 Hz at 1.5 T.

In routine MR imaging, spatial position is assigned along the frequency-encode direction on the basis of resonant frequency. If both water and lipid protons coexist in a voxel, the signal emitted by the lipid protons has a lower frequency than that of the water protons. Consequently, when the system frequency is set to water, *the signal from the lipid protons appears to have arisen from water protons from another voxel in a lower part of the field*. When image intensities are assigned in the final image, therefore, the location of fat protons is spatially mismapped toward the lower part of the readout gradient field.

In clinical imaging, this chemical shift misregistration is manifested as an artifactual white or dark band, one to several pixels in width, most easily seen around the kidneys, around the optic nerves, and at the junction between disks and vertebral bodies (Fig. 6-1). The origin of these chemical shift "bands" is illustrated schematically in Fig. 6-2.

The degree of spatial misregistration between water and fat (and thus the size of the artifact) can be readily computed if one knows the receiver bandwidth (or equivalently, the readout gradient strength and field of view). For example, consider an image with 256 pixels in the frequency-encoding direction that was recorded with a total receiver bandwidth of 32

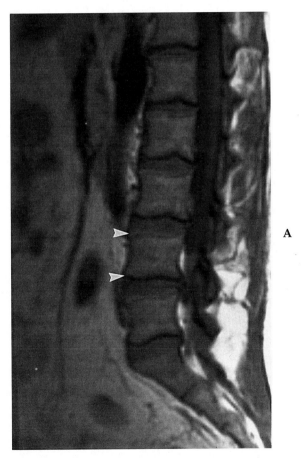

Fig. 6-1. Chemical shift artifacts. **A,** Alternating dark and light bands at the margins of the vertebral bodies. *Continued.*

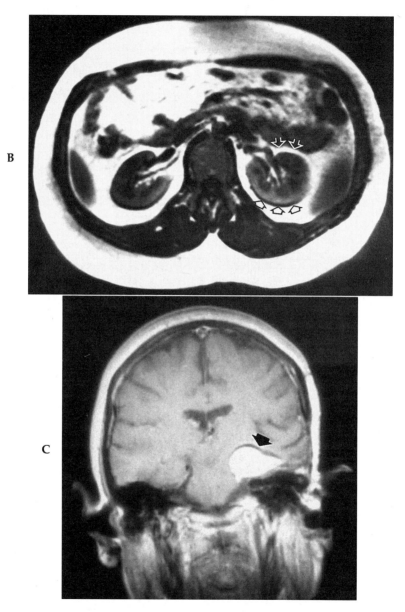

Fig. 6-1 (continued). **B,** Around the edges of organs such as the kidney, imbedded in retroperitoneal fat. **C,** At the junction between normal brain and a fat-containing intracranial dermoid tumor.

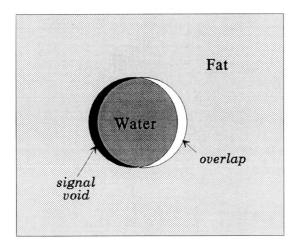

frequency encoding ⟶

Fig. 6-2. Schematic diagram illustrating the origin dark and light bands associated with the chemical shift artifact. A spatial misregistration of fat relative to water signal results in a signal void on one side (*dark band*) and increased signal ("pile up," *light band*) on the other. Note that if the two tissues were switched (i.e., a lump of fat imbedded in water), the positions of the dark and light bands would be reversed.

kHz. The bandwidth per pixel is therefore 32,000/256 = 125 Hz. At 1.5 T, the chemical shift between water and fat is about 225 Hz. In this example, therefore, the size of the chemical shift artifact is calculated to be 225 Hz ÷ 125 Hz/pixel = 1.8 pixels.

If a narrow bandwidth technique is used, the chemical shift artifact is significantly larger. For example, if a receiver bandwidth of 8 kHz is selected, the bandwidth per pixel is only 31 Hz, and the water-fat chemical shift artifact is four times as large, now spanning over 7 pixels. Narrow bandwidth techniques should therefore generally be avoided in locations such as the orbit, where chemical shift artifacts may obscure important interfaces (for instance, that between the optic nerve and orbital fat).

Because the chemical shift artifact is a spatial mismapping of MR signal based on frequency, it is always seen in the frequency-encode direction within a section. Moreover, it should be recognized that in two-dimensional Fourier transform (2DFT) imaging, entire slices are also defined and selected by variations in frequency. Therefore, chemical shift artifacts occur not only within a plane of imaging, but also *between* slices (i.e., in the slice-select direction). Interslice chemical shift artifacts may appear as dark or light "halos" around certain anatomical structures; others are less obvious and result in subtle degradation of image quality.

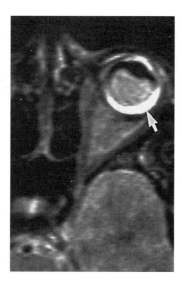

Fig. 6-3. Chemical shift artifact at a water-silicone interface (the eye has been filled with liquid silicone to treat a retinal detachment). Silicone has a chemical shift of 0.3 ppm (compare water at 4.6 and fat at 1.2 ppm).

Finally, one should be aware that chemical shift artifacts not only occur at water-fat interfaces, but may also be seen at the interfaces between any two substances possessing a significant chemical shift. Chemical shift artifacts may therefore also be seen at water-Pantopaque and water-silicone interfaces (Fig. 6-3).

References

Mathews VP, Elster AD, Barker PB et al. Intraocular silicone oil; in vitro and in vivo CT and MR characteristics. AJNR 1993 (in press).

Weinreb JC, Brateman L, Babcock EE et al. Chemical shift artifact in clinical magnetic resonance images at 0.35 T. AJR 145:183, 1985.

| Q 6.02 | Doesn't the chemical shift between water and fat protons also result in a phase shift between them? If this is so, why aren't chemical shift artifacts seen in the phase-encode direction as well? |

It is indeed true that the chemical shift between water and fat protons produces both a frequency shift and a phase shift between the two species.

In routine *spin echo imaging*, however, the resulting extra phase of fat protons relative to water protons does not accumulate from one phase-encoding step to the next. The differential phase shift between water and fat is therefore constant at a given location between successive phase-encoding steps. Since the Fourier transform takes into account the phase *difference* in assigning spatial location to a signal in this direction, no water-fat misregistration occurs along the phase-encoding axis in routine spin echo or gradient echo imaging.

In echo planar imaging (EPI), however, exactly the opposite phenomenon occurs. Here, chemical shift artifacts are minimal in the frequency-encode direction but may be extremely large in the phase-encode direction. The reason for this difference between spin echo and echo planar techniques lies in the way data are collected in the latter (see Q 9.21 for a more complete discussion of EPI).

In EPI all the lines of raw data are collected immediately after a single radiofrequency (RF) excitation. The bandwidth per pixel in the frequency-encode direction is extremely large (i.e., on the order of 2000 Hz), so chemical shift artifacts are not noticeable. In the phase-encode direction, however, the bandwidth per pixel is extremely small (i.e., on the order of 30 Hz), since all the phase-encode lines are acquired in only a few dozen milliseconds. At 1.5 T the fat-water chemical shift is about 225 Hz, and this low bandwidth in the phase-encode direction is translated into a noticeable artifact seven to eight pixels in width. Special corrections and modifications to EPI must be made to minimize the fat signal and eliminate this artifact.

Reference

Szumowski J, Simon JH. Proton chemical shift imaging. In Stark DD, Bradley WG Jr, eds. Magnetic resonance imaging, 2nd ed. St Louis: Mosby–Year Book, 1991, pp 488-490.

Q
6.03

What can one do to eliminate or minimize the chemical shift artifact in routine spin warp imaging?

Once recognized, chemical shift artifacts can generally be "read around" and should not cause major difficulties in image interpretation. If one is trying to detect subtle abnormalities of the optic nerve or small disk herniations in the thoracic spine, however, chemical shift artifacts may be of sufficient size to obscure a lesion completely.

One simple way to work around the chemical shift artifact is to swap the frequency-encode and phase-encode axes before imaging. Doing so will not eliminate the chemical shift artifact but will rotate it to a different anatomical area. Such a strategy may not be successful, however, since it may cause phase wraparound or flow-related artifacts to be shifted over the area of interest instead.

A second strategy is to adjust imaging parameters to reduce the size of the artifact. This goal can be accomplished by increasing the total receiver bandwidth (or equivalently, by increasing the magnitude of the readout gradient).

A final strategy, perhaps the best, is to use some sort of fat suppression technique to reduce the signal from fat and thereby minimize the artifact. Such techniques, including the use of the short TI inversion recovery (STIR) sequence and fat saturation pulses, are discussed in detail in Chapter 9.

Q 6.04	What is a chemical shift artifact of the second kind?

In spin echo (SE) imaging, the signals between water and fat come back into phase at the center of every echo, even though they differ in frequency and are spatially misregistered. In gradient echo (GRE) imaging, however, water and fat protons do not generally come into phase coherence at the center of the echo, since the GRE sequence lacks the 180° refocusing pulse, which accomplishes this task in SE imaging. In a GRE sequence, therefore, fat and water protons go in and out of phase with one another as a function of echo time (TE) (Fig. 6-4). At 1.5 T the period of this alternation is about

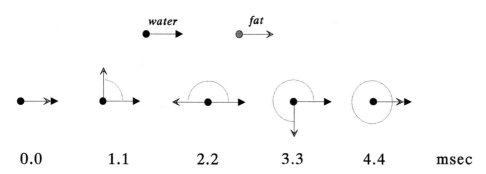

Fig. 6-4. At 1.5 T, fat and water protons go alternately in and out of phase with each other about every 2.2 msec (at 0.5 T, the value is 6.6 msec). In gradient echo imaging, this results in an oscillatory pattern of signal intensity within voxels containing both fat and water protons.

1/225 Hz or 4.4 msec. Therefore, at TE = 2.2, 6.6, 11.0, 15.4 msec, and so on, fat and water fall out of phase with one another in GRE images at 1.5 T. GRE images acquired with TEs near these "magic values" demonstrate chemical shift artifacts of the second kind.

The characteristic appearance of this type of artifact is a sharply defined black rim around objects such as muscle fascicles on GRE images (Fig. 6-5). This artifact arises from boundary pixels that contain both fat and water protons. Since the water and fat in these pixels are out of phase, their signals cancel each other, resulting in a signal void. This is manifest by an eerie black halo along the entire fat-water interface. Notice that since this is a phase cancellation effect, it is not limited to the frequency-encode direction (as is the chemical shift artifact of the first kind) but may be seen in all pixels along a fat-water interface.

Reference

Wehrli FW, Perkins TG, Shimakawa A, Roberts F. Chemical shift–induced amplitude mod-
ulations in images obtained with gradient refocusing. Magn Reson Imaging 5:157, 1987.

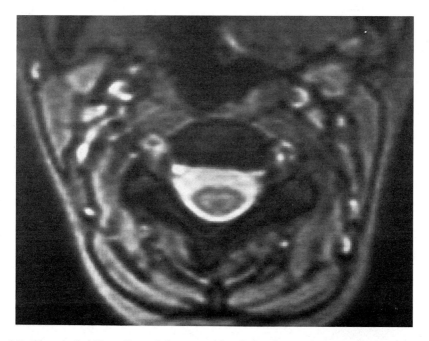

Fig. 6-5. Chemical shift artifact of the second kind. Gradient echo image acquired at 1.5 T with TE = 15.4 msec, which is a "magic value" when fat and water are out of phase. Note the artificially dark borders around muscle fascicles, which result from phase cancellation effects in boundary pixels containing both fat and water.

Q **What is a truncation artifact?**

6.05

Truncation artifacts (also known as ringing, Gibbs, or spectral leakage artifacts) typically appear as multiple parallel lines immediately adjacent to high-contrast interfaces (Fig. 6-6). These artifacts are particularly problematic in spinal imaging, in which they may artifactually widen or narrow the cord or mimic a syrinx.

Truncation artifacts occur as a consequence of using Fourier transforms to reconstruct MR signals into images. In theory, any signal can be represented as an infinite summation of sine waves of different amplitudes, phases, and frequencies (see Q 4.01 for a more detailed explanation of this process). In MR imaging, however, we are restricted to sampling a finite number of frequencies and must therefore approximate the image by using only a relatively few harmonics in its Fourier representation. The Fourier series, then, is cut short or *truncated*, thus the name for this artifact.

If the signal intensity of an object changes gradually in space, only a few Fourier terms are needed, and truncation errors are not evident. At high-contrast interfaces, however, truncation of the Fourier series results in significant artifacts, manifested by variable undershoot and overshoot oscillations (Fig. 6-7). Depending on the number of pixels spanning a high-contrast interface, truncation artifacts may have a variety of forms, including artifactual false widening of the edges at these interfaces or edge enhancement of the interface and distortion of tissues immediately adjacent to the interface. For example, the slightly higher signal seen along the edges of the spinal cord in Fig. 6-6, *B*, is another manifestation of the truncation artifact.

Because truncation artifacts arise as a fundamental consequence of the Fourier representation of an image, they occur in both the phase-encode and frequency-encode directions. However, because fewer samples are usually taken in the phase-encode direction (e.g., 128 or 192), the artifact is usually best seen in this direction. Truncation errors can be minimized by increasing the number of phase-encode steps to 256 or by reducing the field of view. They can never be entirely eliminated, however.

References

Czervionke LF, Czervionke JM, Daniels DL, Haughton VM. Characteristic features of MR truncation artifacts. AJNR 9:815, 1988.

Levy LM, Di Chiro G, Brooks RA et al. Spinal cord artifacts from truncation errors during MR imaging. Radiology 166:479, 1988.

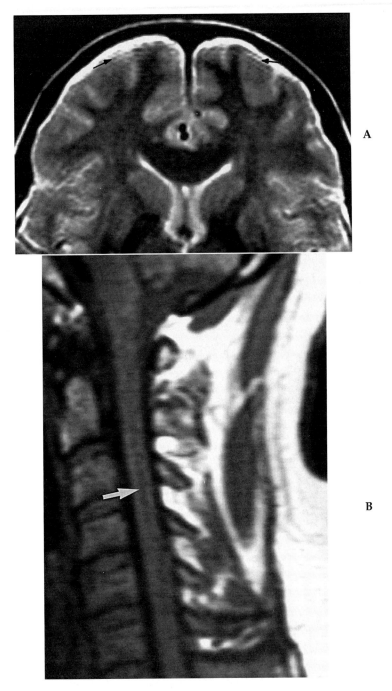

Fig. 6-6. Truncation artifacts. **A,** Multiple fine bands from truncation artifact are seen adjacent to the brain-skull interface. **B,** Truncation artifact in the spinal cord simulating a syrinx (128 × 256 matrix). *Continued.*

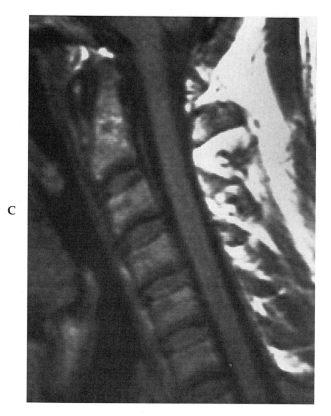

C

Fig. 6-6 (continued). C, After increasing matrix to 256 × 256, the single dark truncation artifact has been replaced by a series of fine bands.

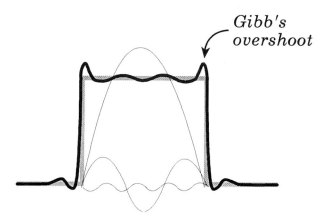

Gibb's overshoot

Fig. 6-7. Truncation (Gibbs) artifacts result from using only a finite number of frequencies in the Fourier representation of a signal. This results in overshoot and undershoot oscillations when sharp borders are encountered in the image.

Q

6.06

What are susceptibility artifacts?

Susceptibility artifacts occur at interfaces between substances with different magnetic susceptibilities. As discussed in Chapter 1, magnetic susceptibility is a fundamental property of matter, resulting primarily from its electronic structure, that serves to either concentrate or disperse the lines of an externally applied magnetic field. When two materials with different magnetic susceptibilities are juxtaposed, a local distortion of the magnetic field exists. This distortion creates dephasing and frequency shifts of nearby protons (and thus artifacts in the MR image).

Since ferromagnetic materials typically have large susceptibilities, field distortions and MR artifacts are prominent around implanted metal objects (e.g., clips, plates, screws). More subtle forms of susceptibility distortions (Fig. 6-8) may be seen at natural interfaces (e.g., trabecular bone, paranasal sinuses, skull base, sella). The shape (diffuse or focal) and intensity (high or low) of the artifact depend on local anatomical relationships as well as the magnitude and direction of the readout gradient (Fig. 6-9).

Susceptibility artifacts may be changed in shape, but not eliminated, by altering the direction of frequency encoding and phase encoding. These artifacts can be minimized by using shorter TE values (less time for dephasing) and by using SE instead of GRE sequences (the 180° refocusing pulse in SE imaging corrects for susceptibility-induced dephasing of stationary protons). Susceptibility artifacts can also be reduced by increasing gradient strength for a given field of view and avoiding narrow bandwidth techniques.

References

Elster AD. Sellar susceptibility artifacts: theory and implications. AJNR 14:129, 1993.

Lüdeke KM, Röschmann P, Tischler R. Susceptibility artefacts in NMR imaging. Magn Reson Imaging 3:329, 1985.

Q

6.07

Why does phase wraparound occur?

Wrap-around, or aliasing, occurs whenever the dimensions of an object exceed the defined field of view (FOV). Although this phenomenon may

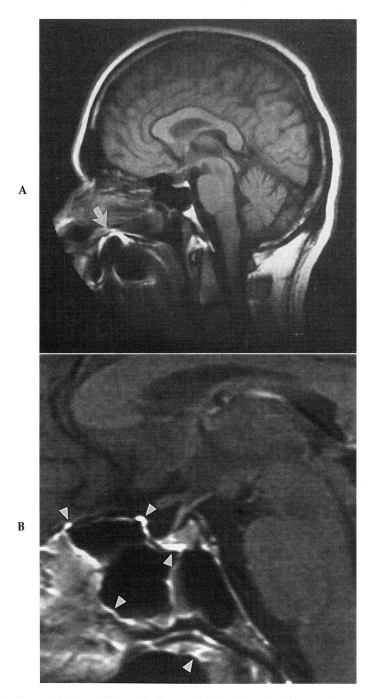

Fig. 6-8. Susceptibility artifacts. **A,** Susceptibility distortion is prominent near metallic orthodontic device *(arrow).* **B,** Natural air-tissue susceptibility artifacts are often seen at the skull base and borders of the paranasal sinuses *(arrowheads).*

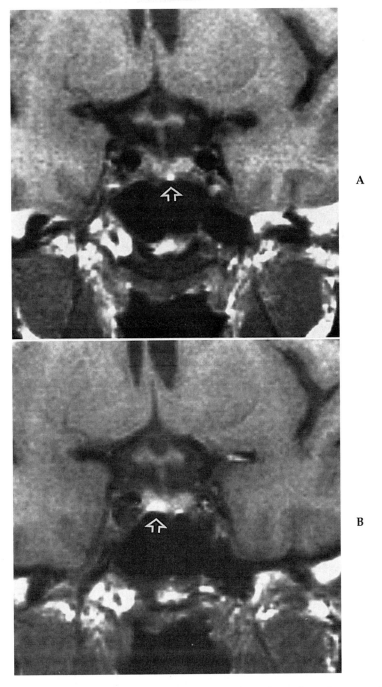

A

B

Fig. 6-9. Shape, size, and intensity of susceptibility artifacts depend on the strength and direction of the readout gradient. The susceptibility artifact at the floor of the sella changes dramatically from **A** to **B** as the direction of the readout gradient is reversed.

occur in the frequency-encode direction (see Q 6.09), it is generally more severe along the phase-encode axis (Fig. 6-10).

The physical basis for this phenomenon is illustrated in Fig. 6-11. Note that for each value of the phase-encoding gradient, a specific number of phase cycles is assigned to cover the FOV. In the first phase-encode step, for example, phase shifts of between 0° and 360° encompass the FOV. Any part of the object that extends beyond the FOV is assigned a phase either less than 0° or greater than 360°. Consider, for example, the subject's left flank in Fig. 6-10; it extends outside the FOV and experiences a phase shift from 361° to 450°. Since at this phase-encoding step all meaningful frequencies have been defined over the range of 0° to 360°, a phase shift of 361° is assigned to the spatial position of 1°, and a shift of 450° is assigned to $450° - 360° = 90°$. The left side of the patient's body therefore is "wrapped around" and spatially mismapped to the opposite (right) side of the image. A similar process wraps the patient's right side around to the left.

Phase wrap-around artifacts may also occur between slices in three-dimensional Fourier transform (3DFT) imaging. In 3DFT (volumetric) imaging, phase encoding is also used to define the individual sections. If the imaged volume extends beyond the FOV in the slab-select direction, a phase wrap-around may occur between slices at the ends of the 3D partition (Fig. 6-12).

The simplest way to eliminate the phase wrap-around artifact is to increase the FOV to encompass the entire anatomical dimension of the subject in that direction. This solution cannot be exercised with impunity, however, since if the FOV is increased, spatial resolution declines. To maintain spatial resolution, therefore, the number of phase-encoding steps must be increased. Phase wrap-around is eliminated, but at the cost of increased imaging time.

As an alternative strategy, the frequency-encoding and phase-encoding axes may be swapped so that the shorter dimension of the subject is oriented in the phase-encode direction. If the FOV is very small, however, even the shorter anatomical dimension of the subject may still exceed the FOV and phase wrap-around still occur. Additionally, switching phase and frequency may introduce different unwanted artifacts over the image (e.g., motion-induced phase ghosts, chemical shift artifacts), thus limiting the usefulness of this simple strategy.

Another group of techniques eliminates phase wrap-around by minimizing the signal from the tissue outside the FOV. These techniques include using a surface coil (which does not detect signals far away from it) and applying saturation pulses outside the FOV (to eliminate the signal from tissues there).

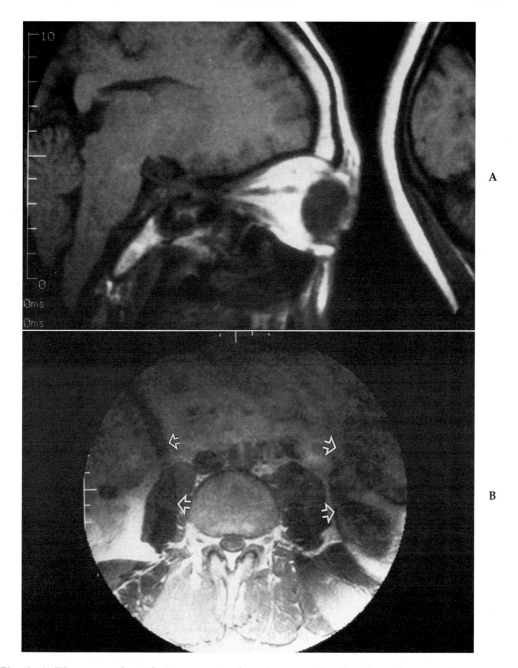

Fig. 6-10. Wrap-around artifact occurs in the phase-encode direction whenever the dimensions of an object exceed the defined field of view. **A,** The back of the head wrapped around to the opposite side. **B,** Both hips are wrapped around on the lumbar spine.

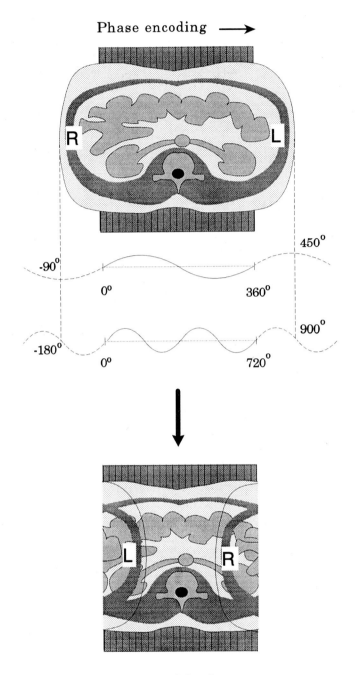

Fig. 6-11. Physical basis for the phase wrap-around artifact. See Q 6.06 for details.

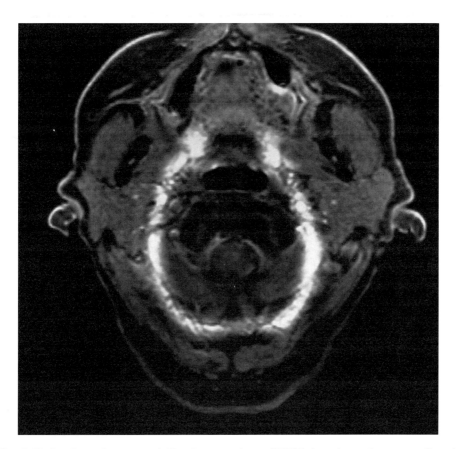

Fig. 6-12. In three-dimensional Fourier transform (3DFT) imaging, phase encoding is performed in the slice-select direction, and phase wraparound artifacts may occur in this direction as well. On this 3DFT head study, the upper part of the brain has been wrapped around to overlie the skull base.

Finally, "no-phase-wrap," "extended matrix," or "antialiasing" software is now available on most commercial scanners, which largely eliminates the phase wrap-around artifact in most cases (see Q 6.08).

Q 6.08	How does "no phase wrap" or "antialiasing" work?

This technique involves four steps, usually performed automatically in scanner software when this option is selected: (1) the FOV is doubled in the phase-encode direction, (2) the number of phase-encoding steps is doubled, (3) the number of excitations is cut in half, and (4) only the middle portion of the reconstructed image is displayed (Fig. 6-13). Steps 1 and 2 maintain spatial resolution at a level identical to that before the "no-phase-wrap" option was selected. Step 3 preserves signal-to-noise ratio (SNR) and imaging time.

Although in general the no-phase-wrap technique may be used without penalty, certain limitations and special considerations apply. First, no-phase-wrap cannot be combined with some specialized multisection techniques (e.g., POMP [see Q 9.10]), which also require doubling the defined FOV and altering phase offsets. Second, since the number of excitations must be halved, the antialiasing technique can be applied without time penalty only to scans in which at least two excitations were originally selected. No-phase-wrap with a single excitation sequence can still be performed but requires the use of partial Fourier ("½-NEX") imaging (see Q 9.11) with a consequent loss in SNR and increase in phase errors.

Finally, the no-phase-wrap technique will not prevent noise and motion-induced phase shifts originating in tissues outside the FOV from propagating into the imaged volume, even though stationary tissues are effectively excluded. For example, a sagittal cervical spine examination phase encoded in a superior to inferior direction may still be degraded by respiratory and cardiac pulsation artifacts, although the heart and chest are not visually wrapped over the spinal image.

| | **Why aren't wrap-around (aliasing) artifacts seen in the frequency-encode direction, too?** |

Wraparound, or aliasing, is a phenomenon fundamental to digital signal processing and can theoretically occur in both the phase-encode and frequency-encode directions. The basis for this phenomenon is illustrated in Fig. 6-14, where a high-frequency signal is inadequately sampled and thereby misinterpreted as a signal of lower frequency. This mismapping of high frequencies into a lower part of the spectrum is known as frequency wraparound or frequency aliasing.

To avoid frequency aliasing, digital sampling of the MR signal must be performed at least twice as rapidly as the highest frequency expected. This critical sampling rate is known as the *Nyquist frequency*. If the signal is sampled less frequently than the Nyquist limit, a misassignment of higher frequencies as lower frequencies will occur.

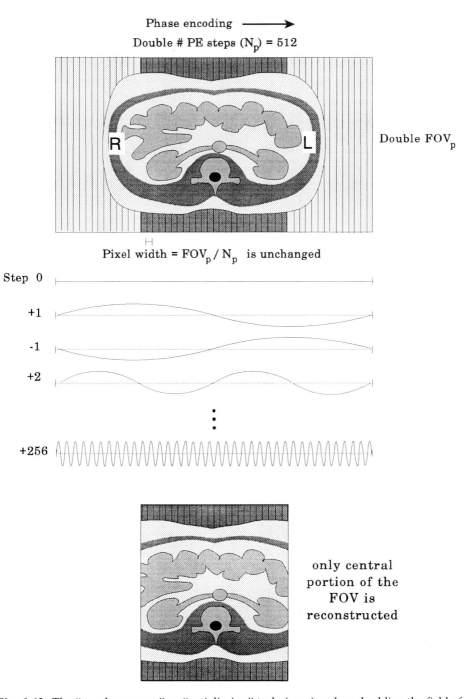

Fig. 6-13. The "no-phase-wrap" or "antialiasing" technique involves doubling the field of view and number of phase-encoding steps, with reconstruction and display of only the central portion of the image. Imaging time and signal-to-noise ratio are maintained by halving the number of excitations.

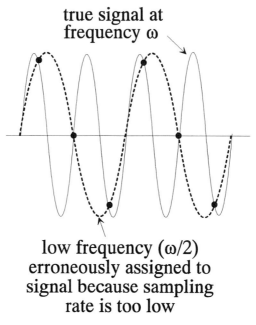

true signal at
frequency ω

low frequency (ω/2)
erroneously assigned to
signal because sampling
rate is too low

Fig. 6-14. Frequency aliasing. See Q 6.09 for details.

Frequency aliasing is not usually a problem in modern clinical MR imaging, since it is largely eliminated by signal oversampling and bandpass filtering before the image is reconstructed. *Oversampling* means that more data measurements of the MR signal are performed than required for image display resolution. In most modern MR scanners, the MR signal is sampled 512 times per echo, even though the display resolution in the frequency-encode direction is usually taken to be 256. Because this task is accomplished by merely increasing the digitizing rate of the sampling circuitry, it imposes no time penalty and occurs "invisibly." In addition to oversampling, the MR signal is also routinely passed through a steep bandpass filter, further eliminating many spurious high-frequency components. As a result of oversampling and filtering, frequency aliasing is essentially imperceptible in modern MR imagers.

Reference

Henkelman RM, Bronskill MJ. Artifacts in magnetic resonance imaging. Rev Magn Reson Med 2:7, 1987.

Q	Why are most motion artifacts (e.g., respiratory, swallowing, flow) propagated in the phase-encode direction instead of in the frequency-encode direction?
6.10	

In 2DFT imaging, considerable disparity exists between sampling times for data collection in the frequency-encode and phase-encode directions. In the frequency-encode direction, all 256 samples of a signal are acquired in the space of a single echo (e.g., over 5 to 25 msec). Conversely, the time to obtain a single sample in the phase-encode direction is on the order of seconds to minutes, since essentially all lines of k-space must be collected to obtain the complete data set for Fourier reconstruction.

Most gross physiological motions (respiration, swallowing, cardiac pulsation) occur over a hundred milliseconds to several seconds. Because these motions are slow in relation to the frequency-encode sampling interval, they typically produce only a small amount of spatial blurring locally in the frequency-encode direction. Conversely, since the phase sampling interval is generally equal to or longer than the period of most physiological motions, artifacts are more prominent in this direction. Furthermore, these artifacts are propagated in the phase-encode direction regardless of whether the physiological motion has occurred in the frequency-encode, phase-encode, or slice-select direction.

Q	Why do motion artifacts sometimes form into discrete ghosts?
6.11	

Discrete "ghost" artifacts may occur along the phase-encode direction whenever the position or signal intensity of imaged structures within the FOV varies or moves in a regular (periodic) fashion. Pulsatile flow of blood or cerebrospinal fluid (CSF), cardiac motion, and respiratory motion are the most important patient-related causes of ghost artifacts in clinical MR imaging (Fig. 6-15). The intensity of these ghost artifacts increases with the amplitude of the periodic motion, as well as with the signal intensity of the moving tissue.

If the motion is nonperiodic (e.g., peristalsis), discrete ghosts are not formed. Instead, diffuse image noise is generated and propagated widely along the phase-encode direction.

The spacing of discrete ghost artifacts in the image depends on the principal direction of motion (along the x, y, or z axis), the magnitude of the displacement, and the periodicity of the motion relative to the

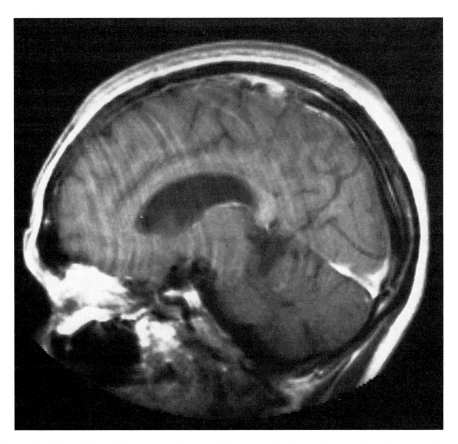

Fig. 6-15. Ghostlike artifacts typically result from periodic motion, such as that associated with pulsatile flow of blood or cerebrospinal fluid. In this case, pulsatile blood flow in the superior sagittal sinus produces a ghosting artifact across the entire brain.

phase-sampling interval. In general, the more rapid the motion, the more widely spaced are the ghosts. For routine 2DFT MR imaging, the interval between successive phase samples is equal to repetition time (TR) times number of excitations (NEX), since repeated excitations are generally performed before incrementing the phase-encode gradient. Ghost artifacts are most closely spaced when the period of motion (TP) equals TR × NEX. Conversely, ghost artifacts are most widely spaced when TP = 2 × TR × NEX.

References

Axel L, Summers RM, Kressel HY, Charles C. Respiratory effects in two-dimensional Fourier transform MR imaging. Radiology 160:795, 1986.

Wood ML, Henkelman RM. MR image artifacts from periodic motion. Med Phys 12:143, 1985.

Q
6.12

How can ghost artifacts be eliminated?

Fortunately, several techniques are available for reducing ghost artifacts. These include (1) physical restraint of body motion, (2) suppression of signal from tissue generating the ghosts, (3) manipulation of imaging parameters, (4) gating, and (5) phase reordering.

Physical restraint of body motion is a simple but effective method for minimizing certain motion-related artifacts. Compression devices (corsets) may be placed around the chest or upper abdomen to limit respiratory excursion and associated artifacts. Papooselike restraints may be useful for infants and small children as an adjunct to sedation. Padding and taping of the neck and extremities may be useful to reduce motion artifacts in surface coil studies of these regions.

A second technique to minimize ghost artifacts is to suppress signal from the moving tissue that causes them. Surface coil imaging may be useful in this regard, since unwanted ghost signals originating in tissues far away from the coil are significantly attenuated. If the ghost signal arises from the motion of abdominal or chest wall fat (which is frequently the case for respiratory artifacts), suppression of this signal with RF saturation bands or by using the STIR technique may be useful. Saturation pulses placed outside the FOV to saturate signal from inflowing blood or CSF may also reduce vascular-related ghost artifacts.

Simple manipulation of imaging parameters may also be helpful. Swapping the frequency-encode and phase-encode axes may serve to rotate the ghosts to a different anatomical area and away from the region of interest. Increasing the number of signal averages also reduces the artifact.

Cardiac or respiratory gating may also be useful to control artifacts from cardiovascular or thoracic motion. These methods require special hardware, however, and often result in an imaging time penalty and restriction of TR to some multiple of the cardiac or respiratory cycle.

Phase-reordering methods (ROPE, COPE, Exorcist, "respiratory comp") seem to be the most practical way at present to reduce respiratory motion artifacts. In routine MR imaging, phase-encoding steps are randomly associated with phases of the respiratory cycle. Phase-reordering techniques assign a specific order to the acquisition of the phase-encoding steps, synchronizing them to consistent times within the respiratory cycle. In the COPE (centrally ordered phase encoding) technique, for example, the phase-encoding gradient amplitude is maximized during end inspiration and minimized during end expiration. Unlike respiratory gating, which may prolong imaging time by 200% to 400%, phase-reordering methods are associated with only a modest time penalty of 10% to 15%, excluding the time needed to fit and calibrate the respiratory bellows.

References

Bailes DR, Gildendale DJ, Bydder GM et al. Respiratory ordered phase encoding (ROPE): a method for reducing respiratory motion artifacts in MR imaging. J Comput Assist Tomogr 9:835, 1985.

Haacke EM, Patrick JL. Reducing motion artifacts in two-dimensional Fourier transform imaging. Magn Reson Imaging 4:359, 1986.

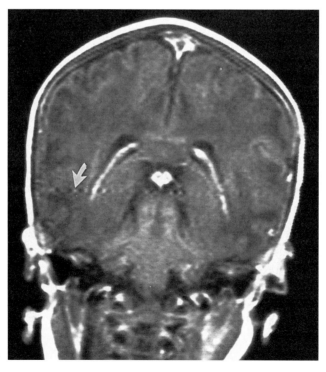

Fig. 6-16. Zipperlike artifact *(arrow)* in the phase-encode direction caused by radiofrequency feedthrough from a pulse oximeter.

Q 6.13 | **We intermittently see zipperlike artifacts in our images. What causes them?**

Because zipperlike bands of spurious signal passing through the image (Fig. 6-16) result from a variety of causes, no single maneuver may correct them all. The most common form of zipper artifact passes through the center of the image and is oriented in the phase-encode direction. This type of zipper artifact results from varying transmitter leakage ("feedthrough") picked up by the receiver system. Perhaps the most common origin of this RF noise is an extraneous source that reaches the receiver coil because the door of the RF-shielded scanner room has not been fully closed. A second common cause is RF emission from anesthesia monitoring equipment (e.g., pulse oximeters) used within the scanner room.

Zipperlike artifacts oriented in the frequency-encode direction are usually caused by stimulated echoes from imperfect slice-selection profiles or improper RF transmitter adjustments. Increasing interslice gap may minimize them, but a call to the service engineer is usually in order.

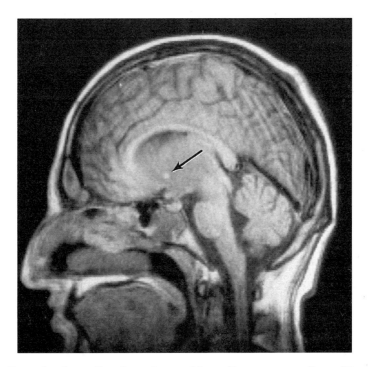

Fig. 6-17. Central point artifact *(arrow)* caused by a direct current offset calibration error.

Reference

Henkelman RM, Bronskill MJ. Artifacts in magnetic resonance imaging. Rev Magn Reson Med 2:7, 1987.

Q
Are there any other common artifacts that we should be aware of?

6.14

I can think of several.

First, there is the *central point artifact*, which appears as either a bright or a dark dot precisely at the center of the image (Fig. 6-17). I have reviewed

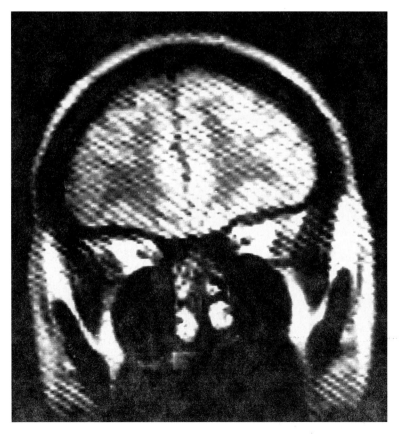

Fig. 6-18. Crisscross or herringbone artifacts are usually caused by a data handling or reconstruction error. These occur sporadically and can usually be corrected by saving the raw data and reconstructing the image again.

MR scans in which this artifact was originally misinterpreted as a multiple sclerosis plaque or a vascular lesion. Don't let this happen to you! The central point artifact results from a constant direct current (DC) offset in the level of receiver voltage of each phase-encoding step. In the early days of MR, this artifact was a common nuisance. Today, however, it is rarely encountered because of the widespread use of RF phase alternation and self-calibrating checks in the scanner circuitry. Occasionally, however, if a DC offset error slips through, the central point artifact may appear in your images. So be prepared.

Another MR artifact one occasionally sees is a crisscross or herringbone artifact (Fig. 6-18). This artifact is generally caused by a data error in processing the Fourier transform. Often, simply reprocessing the raw data removes this artifact and salvages an otherwise unreadable group of images.

Finally, improper calibration of the RF attenuator can result in data clipping and an eerie, phantomlike image with a gray background (see Fig. 3-5). This artifact occurs whenever the attenuator setting is too low and the RF signal saturates (exceeds the upper cutoff level of) the RF amplifier. Careful recalibration and rescanning are the only means of overcoming this artifact.

Reference

Elster AD. Magnetic resonance imaging: a reference guide and atlas. Philadelphia: Lippincott, 1986, p 56.

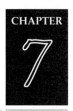
Flow Phenomena and MR Angiography

Because magnetic resonance angiography (MRA) is one of the "hot" new areas in MR development, this entire chapter is devoted to the technique. To understand MRA, however, it is necessary to first review several basic concepts about the physiology of flow and its appearance on routine MR images.

Q 7.01	How is blood flow measured in a vessel?

The total volume of blood that passes a certain point in the vascular tree within a given time is known as the bulk flow and is expressed in units of cubic centimeters per second (cm^3/sec). The average blood velocity (V) equals the bulk flow (Q) divided by the cross-sectional area (A) of the vessel:

$$V = Q/A$$

If A is measured in square centimeters (cm^2), the velocity has units of centimeters per second (cm/sec).

At different points within the lumen of a vessel, however, instantaneous blood velocities vary considerably. Near the vessel wall, where fluidic shearing and frictional forces are greatest, the blood flow is nearly zero. Centrally within the lumen, blood flow is most rapid; peak velocity often exceeds the average velocity by 50%. Instantaneous blood flow at a given point in a vessel also depends on the phase of the cardiac cycle in which it is measured. In the proximal aorta, the direction of blood flow even reverses between systole and diastole.

References

Potchen EJ, Haacke EM, Siebert JE, Gottschalk A, eds. Magnetic resonance angiography: concepts and applications. St Louis: Mosby–Year Book, 1993. (A newly published and comprehensive textbook.)

Turski P. Vascular magnetic resonance imaging. Signa applications guide. Vol III. GE Medical Systems Catalogue #E8804DB, 1990, pp 3-5. (This excellent monograph, available through GE sales representatives, is the best place to start reading about general flow phenomena and MRA.)

Q 7.02	What usual blood velocities exist in the human vascular tree?

Normal human peak systolic blood flow velocities vary with age, cardiac output, and anatomical site. The ascending aorta has the highest peak velocities; typical values are 150 to 175 cm/sec. Flow in the distal aorta and iliac vessels slows to 100 to 150 cm/sec whereas peak velocities in the proximal carotid, brachial, and superficial femoral arteries are about 80 to 120 cm/sec. Intracranially, peak velocities of the middle and anterior cerebral arteries are approximately 40 to 70 cm/sec, whereas those in the vertebral-basilar system are only 30 to 50 cm/sec. Venous velocities are generally less than 20 cm/sec. Conversely, in certain pathological conditions such as arteriovenous fistulas, velocities up to 400 cm/sec may be recorded.

Q 7.03	What is the difference between laminar flow, turbulent flow, and vortex flow?

Laminar flow refers to a predictable distribution of flow velocities in layers (laminae) that parallel the vessel wall. This form of flow is idealized but is nevertheless a fairly good approximation of the flow in medium-sized and small-sized blood vessels throughout the human circulatory system. Theoretically, the distribution of velocities in a perfectly straight, non-

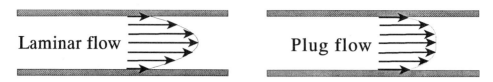

Fig. 7-1. Laminar and plug flow. Laminar flow has a parabolic velocity profile, whereas plug flow is flattened.

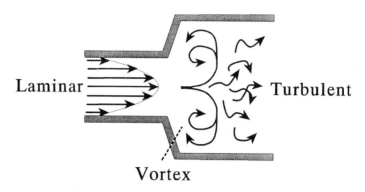

Fig. 7-2. Transition from laminar to turbulent flow at a vascular dilatation. Also note swirling vortex (eddy current) flow in the "corners."

branching vessel with nonpulsatile flow should be parabolic in cross section (Fig. 7-1), with peak velocities at the center of the lumen. In real vessels, however, the flow profile is usually more blunted because of elasticity and pulsatility effects, even though the general laminar pattern may be maintained. When the flow profile becomes flattened in this form with a nearly uniform distribution of velocities across the lumen, the term *plug flow* is sometimes applied.

Turbulent flow is a chaotic form of fluid transport in which velocity components randomly fluctuate (Fig. 7-2). Turbulence takes place when blood velocities exceed a critical threshold or when vascular morphology creates conditions that disrupt the laminar flow state. In the human circulatory system, turbulent flow is seen in the aorta, in the region of vascular bifurcations, and distal to areas of stenosis.

In ideal fluids, turbulence can be predicted on the basis of the calculated value of a dimensionless parameter known as the Reynold's number *(Re)*:

$$Re = \rho dV / \eta$$

where ρ and η are the fluid's density and viscosity, d is the diameter of the vessel, and V is the flow velocity. Values of *Re* less than 2000 predict that flow will be laminar, whereas values greater than 2500 usually indicate that flow will be turbulent.

Vortex flow refers to localized swirling or stagnant blood flow that has separated from the central streamlines within a vessel (Fig. 7-2). Such vortices, also called *flow eddies*, frequently occur at vascular bifurcations and distal to areas of stenosis. Unlike turbulent regions, areas of vortex flow are composed of slowly moving currents and streamlines that are not random but are often countercurrent to the main flow direction. Both turbulent flow and vortex flow create problems for MR angiography.

Reference

Listerud J, Cohen IM. Overview of flow hemodynamics. Neuroimaging Clin North Am 2:719, 1992.

Q 7.04	**How can one predict whether a certain vessel will appear bright or dark on MR images?**

Experienced radiologists generally become familiar with the expected appearances of normal blood vessels on their own scanners when consistent imaging parameters are used. At times they may even be capable of diagnosing subtle disorders of flow by using pattern recognition. However, no radiologist, even a world "expert," can consistently predict or even fully explain the complex signals observed within any vessel, given an arbitrary set of imaging parameters. The reason for this uncertainty is that the appearance of flowing blood on MR images depends in a complex and nonintuitive fashion on both the details of the pulse sequence employed and the physical characteristics of flow.

Technical factors affecting the appearance of flowing blood include the type of pulse sequence (spin echo, gradient echo, inversion recovery), repetition time (TR), echo time (TE), and flip angle (α). The use of flow compensation (gradient moment nulling), saturation pulses, and cardiac gating also has profound effects. Additionally, even small changes in slice thickness, interslice gap, number of slices, or slice excitation order may have radical effects on the appearance of normal blood vessels at MR imaging. Marked variations in the appearance of flow may also exist between different brands of scanners run with otherwise identical user-specified parameters.

Physical characteristics of flow are also important determinants of a vessel's appearance on MR images. These characteristics include not only flow direction and average velocity, but also acceleration, pulsatility, and the distribution of velocities across the vessel. The internal "structure" of the flow is important, since differences are noted between laminar, vortex, and turbulent patterns. No wonder even sophisticated computer programs are not yet fully able to predict the wide spectrum of normal vascular appearances encountered on MR images.

Notwithstanding these uncertainties, several general principles can be derived concerning the appearance of flow on MR images:

1. Rapid or turbulently flowing fluids generally have low signal on conventional spin echo (SE) images, resulting in a *flow void*.

2. Conversely, slowly flowing blood or cerebrospinal fluid (CSF) generally appears bright on conventional SE images, a phenomenon formerly called *paradoxical enhancement*.

3. Fresh blood flowing into a volume of tissue results in high signal in vessels within the end slices of a multisection acquisition; this is a time-of-flight effect called *flow-related enhancement* or simply the *entry phenomenon*.

4. Saturation pulses applied outside the field of view reduce or eliminate the entry phenomenon, making these vessels dark.

5. The use of gradient moment nulling (flow compensation) gradients results in increased signal within veins and smaller arteries, but faster flow in larger arteries still demonstrates flow voids.

6. Cardiac gating may restore signal not only to small vessels, but to larger ones as well.

7. Two different flow-related signal changes may be observed when trains of evenly spaced (i.e., TE = 30/60/90/120) spin echoes are employed. Loss of signal occurs after odd-numbered (30, 90) echoes (*odd echo dephasing*), whereas increased signal is seen on even-numbered (60, 120) echoes (*even echo rephasing*).

8. Gadolinium contrast shortens the T1 of blood and generally increases the signal from all vessels.

These concepts are summarized in Table 7-1 and are further explained in other questions within this chapter.

References

Axel L. Blood flow effects in magnetic resonance imaging. AJR 143:1167, 1984.

Elster AD. Cranial magnetic resonance imaging. New York: Churchill Livingstone, 1988, pp 11-12.

TABLE 7-1. Factors Affecting the MR Signal Observed in Blood Vessels	
Decreased Intravascular Signal	Increased Intravascular Signal
High velocity	Low velocity
Turbulent or vortex flow	Laminar flow
Saturation pulses	Gradient moment nulling
Odd echo dephasing	Even echo rephasing
Multislice acquisition	Single-slice acquisition
Flow within plane of imaging	Flow perpendicular to plane of imaging
Slices deep within imaged volume	Slices at ends of imaged volume
	Cardiac gating
	Gadolinium

Q 7.05   What are time-of-flight effects?

Time-of-flight (TOF) effects refer to signal variations resulting from the motion of protons flowing into or out of an imaging volume during a given pulse sequence. In both SE and gradient echo (GRE) imaging, inflow of spins results in increased signal; this phenomenon is known as *flow-related enhancement*. Conversely, outflow of spins may result in decreased signal intensity, a phenomenon known as *high-velocity signal loss.*

To understand flow-related enhancement, one should recognize that the slab of tissue contained within an imaged volume is repeatedly subjected to radiofrequency (RF) pulses throughout the imaging process. These RF pulses repeatedly flip the longitudinal magnetization of all tissue (including blood) contained within the imaging volume into the transverse plane. This process, known as *saturation*, results in a progressive decrease in the tissue signal until a steady state is reached between the longitudinal recovery of the tissue and the action of these RF pulses. Fresh blood flowing into the imaged volume has not been subjected to these RF pulses and is therefore fully magnetized (unsaturated). When a bolus of this fresh blood enters a slice and is subjected to its first set of RF pulses, the signal it emits is significantly stronger than that of the tissue that has remained within the slab. A "paradoxical" flow-related enhancement of this inflowing blood is then observed (Fig. 7-3).

Flow-related enhancement is more likely to be encountered at the end slices of a multislice acquisition. If the flow is sufficiently rapid, fresh blood

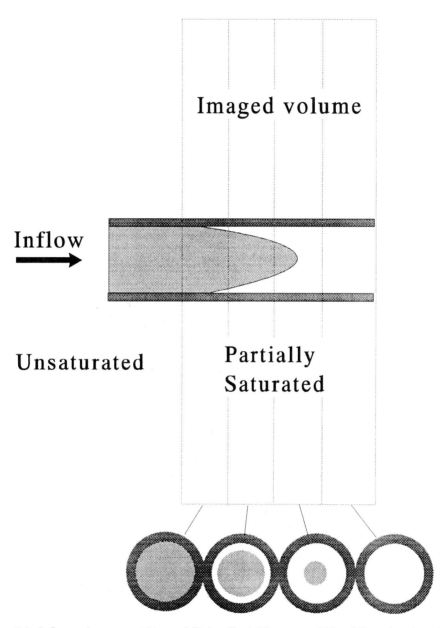

Fig. **7-3.** Inflow enhancement (time-of-flight effect). Unsaturated blood flows into imaging volume, which has been partially saturated by the action of multiple previous radiofrequency pulses. The signal from the new blood is paradoxically higher than one would expect as a result of this inflow phenomenon. As the flow profile penetrates further into the imaged volume, only the higher velocities at the center of the lumen demonstrate this enhancement.

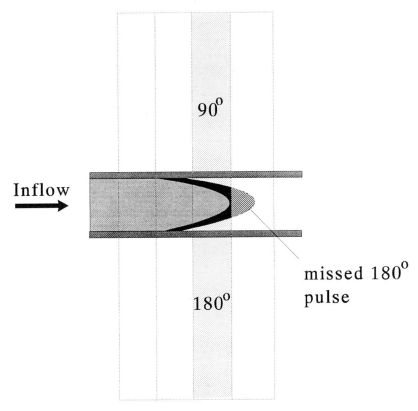

Fig. 7-4. Time-of-flight (TOF) signal loss. Moving bolus of blood must receive both 90° and 180° pulses to emit a signal. If part of the blood moves out of slice before receiving both pulses *(hatched area)*, a TOF signal loss occurs.

may penetrate several slices into the imaged volume before it becomes partially saturated. Accordingly, flow-related enhancement may be observed not only at the end slices but sometimes several slices deep into the imaged volume.

High-velocity signal loss is a TOF effect in which spins flow out of a slice before they are stimulated by both 90° and 180° pulses (Fig. 7-4). This phenomenon occurs only in SE imaging in which a slice-selective 180° refocusing pulse is used. It does not occur in GRE imaging because the gradient used for echo formation is not slice selective. High-velocity signal loss is therefore most prominent on long TE SE images, since long TEs provide a greater opportunity for spins to flow out of the slice between the 90° and 180° pulses.

References

Bradley WG, Waluch V. Blood flow: magnetic resonance imaging. Radiology 154:443, 1985.

Wehrli FW. Time-of-flight effects in MR imaging of flow. Magn Reson Med 14:187, 1990.

Q
7.06

What are spin phase effects?

Spin phase effects refer to changes in precession angle (phase) that protons undergo when they move within a magnetic field gradient. Normally, gradients are applied to produce spatial encoding of the MR signal. In this way, signals coming from stationary tissue in different parts of the subject have a unique "phase signature," and their exact location can be decoded and correctly assigned to a point in the MR image. If the proton changes position while these gradients are applied, however, it will gain or lose phase compared with stationary tissue. In flowing blood, the MR signal changes resulting from this process are termed *spin phase effects*.

To gain some appreciation for the magnitude of spin phase effects, let us calculate directly the phase gained by a proton moving through a magnetic field gradient (Fig. 7-5). For simplicity, we will assume that the proton starts

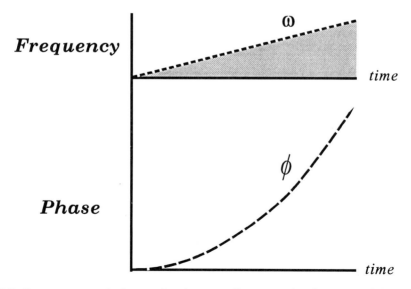

Fig. 7-5. For constant velocity motion in a gradient, angular frequency (ω) increases linearly with time, whereas phase shift (ϕ) increases quadratically.

at magnet isocenter (position $x = 0$) and moves at constant velocity (v) for time (t) in the direction of the gradient (which has constant magnitude G). Since the proton is moving at constant velocity within a constant gradient, its resonant offset frequency (ω) will be a linear function of time and is given by

$$\omega = \gamma Gx = \gamma Gvt$$

Because angular frequency (ω) is merely the differential change in phase with respect to time $(d\phi/dt)$ (see Q 1.16 for an explanation), the phase shift of the proton can be written

$$\phi = \int \omega dt = \int \gamma Gvt \; dt = \gamma Gv \int tdt = \tfrac{1}{2} \gamma Gvt^2$$

This equation thus demonstrates an important (but nonintuitive) concept: the phase shift experienced by a moving spin is proportional to its velocity, the strength of the applied gradient, and the *square* of the length of time it moves within that gradient.

Reference

von Schulthess GV, Higgins CB. Blood flow imaging with MR: spin-phase phenomena. Radiology 157:687, 1985.

Q 7.07 **Why do GRE pulse sequences accentuate the signals from flowing blood and CSF?**

When appropriate imaging parameters are used, GRE sequences generate a strong signal from moving spins, and in this way highlight flowing blood or CSF, making GRE-based sequences the backbone of most MRA techniques. GRE sequences accentuate signals from flowing fluids for three principal reasons.

First, when sequential mode acquisition (rather than interleaved multislice mode) is employed, each section behaves as an "entry slice" and demonstrates flow-related (inflow) enhancement. This statement is true for any flip angle, as long as the sequence is gradient or RF spoiled or the TR value is long enough to minimize steady-state effects.

For steady-state GRE sequences (e.g., GRASS/FISP), flow sensitivity can be increased by using moderate-to-large flip angles. Large flip angles accentuate the signal from flowing blood or CSF for two reasons: (1) they cause more saturation of stationary tissue, and when unsaturated spins flow in, a greater contrast between moving and static tissue can be appreciated; and (2) large flip angles produce signal intensity differences proportional to T2/T1, a ratio that is higher in CSF, blood, and other fluids than for solid tissues.

The second factor increasing the flow sensitivity of GRE imaging concerns the nonselectivity of the refocusing mechanism. In routine SE imaging, at least part of the reason for flow-related signal loss is that spins move out of the section between the 90° and 180° (refocusing) pulses. In GRE imaging the refocusing is done by means of a gradient reversal that is not slice selective. This nonselective refocusing does *not* result in hyperintensity of incoming spins, however; it merely prevents them from experiencing TOF signal losses.

Finally, relatively short TEs are often used in conjunction with GRE techniques to minimize T2* dephasing. Because these short TEs also minimize flow-related signal losses, they accentuate the appearance of the flowing fluid.

Reference

Atlas SW, Mark AS, Fram EK, Grossman RI. Vascular intracranial lesions: applications of gradient-echo MR imaging. Radiology 169:455, 1988.

| Q | How is slow flow distinguished from thrombus on MR |
| 7.08 | images? |

This is a common problem that comes up at least once a week at our institution. Fortunately, there are usually clues on routine imaging sequences, as well as special techniques that may help you resolve this dilemma.

Clues on Routine Imaging

The first step in differentiating between slow flow and thrombus is to look carefully at the area in question on all imaging sequences. It is particularly helpful if the same pulse sequence has been used in two different planes. With slow flow, the intravascular signal often changes when different imaging planes have been used; thrombus has the same intensity regardless of the plane.

A second clue from routine imaging is to compare the signal of the questionable vessel on both T1-weighted and T2-weighted images. Flow enhancement usually fades as TE is increased; thrombus is often of intermediate or high signal on all sequences. (If gradient moment nulling was used on the long TE image, however, this trick will not work.)

Is the abnormal intravascular signal maximal at the end slice, and does it fade out as one moves inward? Chances are you are dealing with inflow enhancement rather than thrombus.

Is there any evidence of phase artifacts (ghosting) adjacent to the vessel? (You may have to rewindow the image and look in the air outside the patient to see it.) If you do see ghosting, some flow must be present.

Does the area in question get brighter with gadolinium? Although gadolinium may diffuse into a clot, seeing a significantly brighter signal after contrast administration supports the diagnosis of vascular patency. However, since tumor thrombi may enhance vividly with gadolinium, contrast enhancement will not aid much in the differential diagnosis in this scenario.

Special Techniques to Resolve the Issue

If MRA is available, we usually first try a two-dimensional (2D) phase contrast technique with a low velocity-encoding (VENC) gradient (e.g., 20 cm/sec). Slow flow often becomes immediately apparent when this technique is used. Very slow flow may still be missed, however.

In my experience, TOF MRA has not been particularly useful in distinguishing acute thrombus from flow. Both may appear bright (thrombus because of methemoglobin, flow because of true flow), and the maximum intensity projection registers signal from both sources.

Another simple technique is to apply a presaturation band upstream from the site of suspected thrombosis. The signal from thrombus is unaffected by this maneuver; flow signal is reduced or eliminated.

If the necessary software is available, narrow saturation bands may also be used for bolus tagging. If the bolus moves, flow is present.

If you have the appropriate software, make a phase map of the image from the raw data. Flowing blood, unlike thrombus, has a higher or lower signal than the background on such phase maps.

It may be helpful to obtain a single-slice GRE image using parameters that you know normally produce high signal in flowing vessels on your scanner. We usually try a 2D Fourier transform (2DFT) SPGR 30/5/35° sequence or a 2DFT GRASS 30/5/90° sequence angled perpendicular to the axis of the vessel.

Even without these "fancy" pulse sequences, you can usually solve the flow/thrombus riddle if you are clever. Try the following:

1. Repeat the T1-weighted or T2-weighted images using a different plane of section than in the original. Slow flow may change its appearance, but thrombus will not.

2. Repeat the sequences with and without gradient moment nulling. Flow may change in appearance, thrombus will not.

3. Try a T2-weighted sequence with multiple symmetrical echoes (e.g., 30/60/90/120), and look carefully for subtle signs of even echo rephasing or odd echo dephasing (which may be present with flow). Use standard scanner software to compute the T2 value within the vessel (nearly every commercial scanner has this software, although most people do not know how to use it). A negative value suggests flow; a positive value, thrombosis.

Q	Please explain even echo rephasing.
7.09	

Even echo rephasing is a flow phenomenon observed in SE images in which multiple symmetrical echoes (e.g., 30/60/90/120) have been employed. For blood flowing at constant velocity in such an environment, it has been observed that phase dispersion is lower on the even-numbered echoes (i.e., 60/120) than on the odd echoes (i.e., 30/90). The absolute increase in flow signal on the second and fourth echoes is called *even echo rephasing*; the loss in signal on the first and third echoes is called *odd echo dephasing*. The gradient causing this echo modulation is the frequency-encoding gradient. Thus, this phenomenon is typically seen in vessels flowing *within* an imaging plane and having some component of their flow in the frequency-encode direction.

To explain why even echo rephasing and odd echo dephasing occur, it is necessary to make use of the fact developed in Q 7.06 that for constant velocity flow through a constant gradient, total phase shift increases quadratically with time *(t)*. In other words:

$$\phi = Kt^2$$

where $K = \frac{1}{2} \gamma Gv$ is a constant when velocity and gradient strength are also constant.

This quadratic dependence of total phase gain on time is shown in Fig. 7-6. This figure illustrates several useful concepts that are helpful in understanding even echo rephasing. Note that after the 1st, 2nd, 3rd, and 4th gradient intervals, each of duration *T*, the phase has increased quadratically to KT^2, $4KT^2$, $9KT^2$, and $16KT^2$, respectively. The *incremental* phase contributions of the 1st, 2nd, 3rd, and 4th gradient intervals are therefore KT^2, $3KT^2$, $5KT^2$, and $7KT^2$, respectively.

Using these calculated incremental phase contributions from each

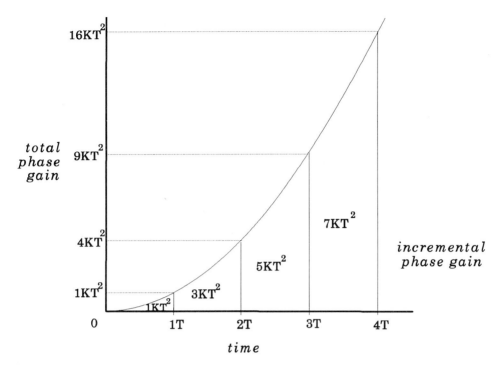

Fig. 7-6. Details of quadratic phase gain with time. Note that *incremental* phase gain per unit time T has a simple pattern ($1KT^2$, $3KT^2$, $5KT^2$, and so on).

block of the gradient, we now can calculate what the phase should be at each point in a multiple SE protocol (Fig. 7-7). Let us now consider the action of the 180° pulses, which invert the level of accumulated phase existing immediately before the pulse. After block 1 but before the 180° pulse, the total accumulated phase is KT^2. Immediately after the 180° pulse, the total phase has been inverted to $-KT^2$. The next block adds $3KT^2$ of phase, after which the total phase at the center of the first echo is $2KT^2$ (i.e., $-KT^2 + 3KT^2$). Thus the first echo has an appreciable phase dispersion because of flow. This is the origin of odd echo dephasing.

Continuing, we see that the readout gradient for the first echo contains another block, which adds another $5KT^2$ of phase. After this block and immediately before the next 180° pulse, the total phase has reached $2KT^2 + 5KT^2 = 7KT^2$. The 180° pulse inverts this phase, so immediately after the 180° pulse, the total phase is $-7KT^2$. To get to the center of the second echo, we must add the incremental phase contribution of the 4th block, which we have previously computed to be $7KT^2$. The total phase at the center of the second echo is therefore $-7KT^2 + 7KT^2 = 0$. In other words, moving spins have come back into phase at the center of the second echo. This is the origin of even echo rephasing.

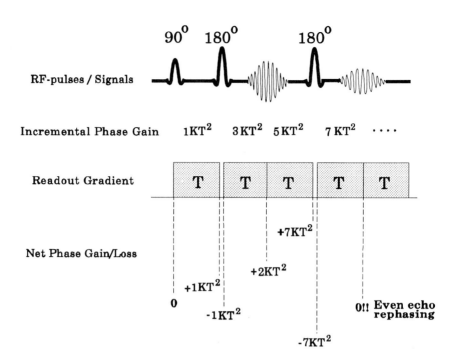

Fig. 7-7. Even echo rephasing. See Q 7.09 for details.

Although this simplified analysis assumes that the gradient pulses are applied back to back, the same results can be demonstrated even when the gradients are spaced out, as they normally are on routine imaging.

Reference

Waluch V, Bradley WG Jr. NMR even echo rephasing in slow laminar flow. J Comput Assist Tomogr 8:594, 1984.

Q
7.10

Please explain how gradient moment nulling works.

Gradient moment nulling (GMN), also known as flow compensation ("flow comp"), gradient motion rephasing (GMR), or motion artifact suppression technique (MAST), operates according to the same principles as even echo rephasing. Please review Q 7.09 and be sure you understand even echo rephasing before you tackle GMN.

In GMN, additional gradient lobes are added before signal readout to

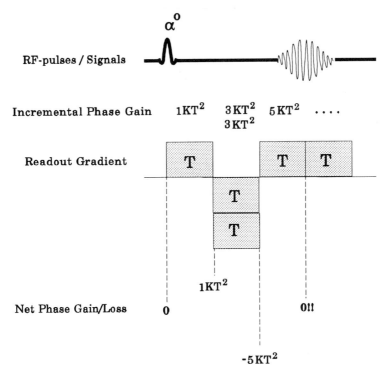

Fig. 7-8. Gradient moment nulling. See Q 7.10 for details.

compensate *in advance* for motion-induced dephasing at the time of the echo. As a simple example, let us analyze the velocity-compensated GRE sequence shown in Fig. 7-8. Note that the readout gradient has a more complex appearance than in the usual GRE sequence (compare with Fig. 5-1). These additional gradient blocks ("lobes") impart to this sequence its flow compensation properties.

First note that for stationary spins, the additional gradient lobes have no net effect. For stationary spins, each lobe adds a constant amount of phase. Since there are two positive-going and two negative-going lobes before the center of the echo, their net effect is zero.

To analyze what happens to a spin moving at constant velocity, we will do an incremental phase calculation as we did in Q 7.09. After the first block, the phase should again be KT^2. The incremental phase contribution from the two blocks that compose the second lobe is $2 \times (-3KT^2) = -6KT^2$. The net phase of the spins immediately after the double block is therefore $KT^2 - 6KT^2 = -5KT^2$. Finally, the first readout block contributes its incremental $+5KT^2$, yielding a net phase of zero at $t = TE$. By adding these extra gradient blocks, we have compensated or corrected for phase dispersions attributable to velocity.

Once again, we have used a simplified scheme in which the blocks were back to back and in a 1:2:1 ratio. Many other variations are possible, including making the gradient lobes smaller and putting spaces between them. It is also possible to add still more lobes to compensate not only for flows with constant velocities, but also for those with constant accelerations and even higher orders of motion. Additionally, flow compensation need not be limited to the frequency-encode direction; it is possible to design sequences with GMN along the slice-select and phase-encode directions as well.

Today, GMN techniques are widely used and available on all MR scanners. The principal limitations of these sequences are that (1) the minimum TE is lengthened because time is needed to fit in the extra gradient lobes; (2) stresses on the imaging gradients are increased, limiting field of view or slice thickness for a given TR; and (3) artifacts caused by eddy currents may be induced by the rapid gradient switching required.

References

Haacke EM, Lenz GW. Improving MR image quality in the presence of motion by using rephasing gradients. AJR 148:1251, 1987.

Pattany PM, Phillips JJ, Chiu LC, et al. Motion artifact suppression technique (MAST) for MR imaging. J Comput Assist Tomogr 11:369, 1987.

Q 7.11	**Please explain why the refocused signal from flowing blood may be spatially misregistered and how the direction of flow can be determined on an MR image.**

In routine SE imaging a pixel is spatially encoded by both phase and frequency. This process is not instantaneous, and in general, phase encoding is performed first. If a spin moves between the times of phase encoding and frequency encoding, its apparent position in the image is artifactually displaced from its true position. This phenomenon is shown in Fig. 7-9.

Spatial misregistration of flow is most prominent for vessels lying within the plane of imaging. It is accentuated by increased TE, since this increases the interval between phase encoding and frequency readout.

For most sequences it is possible to predict the direction of flow when a flow misregistration artifact is noted. One simply looks to see on which side of the vessel the artifact appears in relation to the frequency-encode

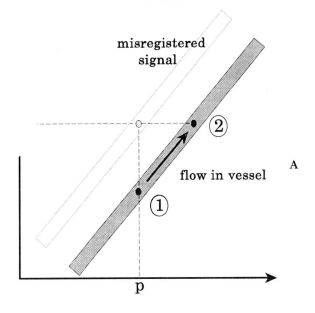

misregistered signal

(2)

flow in vessel

(1)

p

A

phase encoding gradient

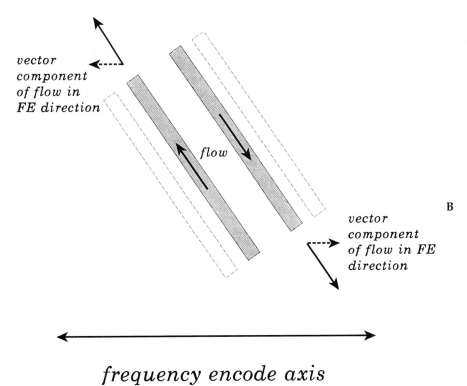

vector component of flow in FE direction

flow

vector component of flow in FE direction

B

frequency encode axis

Fig. 7-9. For legend, see p. 180.

Continued.

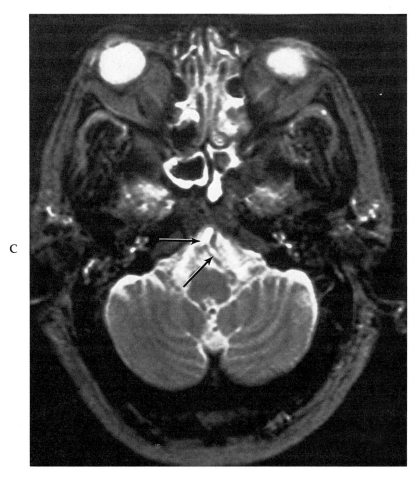

C

Fig. 7-9 (continued). Spatial misregistration of vascular flow on MR images. **A,** The effect originates because in spin echo imaging, phase encoding and frequency encoding are performed at different times. A spin at 1 is first encoded to phase position p. If it then flows to point 2, it is frequency encoded to frequency position f. The final mapping to point p,f is spatially misregistered from the true vascular position. **B,** Direction of flow can be predicted in an MR image by noticing the position of the spatial misregistration relative to the frequency-encode direction. The misregistered signal is always displaced toward the side of the vessel having a vector component of flow in the frequency-encode direction. **C,** Spatial misregistration artifact *(arrowheads)* in the vertebral basilar system.

axis. The artifact will lie on the side of the vessel where there is a vector component of flow. From this information the flow direction can bepredicted in nearly all cases. One should be cautioned, however, that when certain gradient structures or imaging techniques are used, this appearance may be reversed. Despite this limitation, the flow displacement artifact sign is extremely useful in routine imaging, particularly when a vascular malformation is encountered.

Reference

Larson TC III, Kelly WM, Ehman RL, Wehrli FW. Spatial misregistration of vascular flow during MR imaging of the CNS: cause and clinical significance. AJNR 11:1041, 1990.

Q 7.12	What is the difference between time-of-flight and phase contrast MR angiography?

Although a wide variety of MRA sequences are offered by different manufacturers, all can generally be classified as one of two types: time of flight (TOF) or phase contrast (PC). Each technique may be performed in either the 2DFT or the 3DFT mode and may be combined with other imaging options, such as saturation pulses, magnetization transfer pulses, gradient moment nulling, or cardiac gating. Each technique has distinct advantages and disadvantages, as discussed here and summarized in Table 7-2.

TOF MRA is based on a conventional 2DFT or 3DFT GRE sequence with gradient moment nulling. A presaturation pulse is often applied above or below each slice to reduce signal from overlying arteries or veins. A moderate-to-large flip angle (e.g., 30° to 60°) is used to maximize contrast between stationary tissue and blood. Short TE values (< 5 to 7 msec) are preferred to minimize signal loss from phase dispersion.

TOF MRA is based on the principle of flow-related enhancement (discussed in Q 7.05). Blood flowing into a slice paradoxically appears brighter than stationary tissue because it has not become saturated by multiple previous RF pulses. Maximum enhancement of flow occurs when the vessel is perpendicular to the plane of imaging. TOF techniques are thus somewhat insensitive to in-plane flow. Also, because of saturation effects, maximum slab thickness may be limited.

TOF techniques rely principally on RF pulses to saturate stationary tissue and to increase contrast to the entering flows. However, some substances with short T1 values (fat, methemoglobin, gadolinium) may be incompletely saturated and "shine through" on the maximum intensity projection (MIP) reconstruction.

PC MRA makes use of velocity-induced phase shifts to distinguish flowing blood from stationary tissue. Although several pulse sequence variations are possible, nearly all are GRE techniques that use bipolar (flow-encoding) gradients along one or more axes. The fundamental flow principle underlying this strategy is that stationary spins experience no net phase shift by this combination of positive and negative gradients, whereas spins moving with constant velocity experience a phase shift proportional

TABLE 7-2. Advantages and Disadvantages of Time-of-Flight (TOF) and Phase Contrast (PC)

MRA Technique	Advantages	Disadvantages
2D TOF	Sensitivity to slow flow	Insensitivity to in-plane flow
	Short acquisition times	Patient motion may create spatial misregistration
		High signal from fat or blood may mimic flow
3D TOF	High spatial resolution	Insensitivity to slow flow; venous anatomy especially poor
	Sensitivity to medium and fast flow	Saturation effects limit maximum slab thickness
	Ability to obtain very short TEs	High signal from fat or blood may mimic flow
	High signal-to-noise ratio	
2D PC	Short imaging times allow testing of multiple velocity encodings (VENCs)	Patient motion may create spatial misregistration
	By adjusting VENC, user can emphasize arteries or veins	Large voxel size results in increased intravoxel phase dispersion
	Can quantitate velocity and direction of flow	
3D PC	Can be made sensitive to various velocities through adjustment of VENC	Optimum VENC often unknown in advance
	Background suppression excellent even with fat, blood, or gadolinium nearby	Sensitivity to patient motion
		Imaging times relatively long
	Saturation effects minimal over large volumes	Turbulence may produce greater signal loss on PC than TOF

to flow velocity, amplitude of the bipolar gradient, and time interval between the gradient lobes. The amplitude of the bipolar gradient determines the degree of velocity encoding (VENC); by adjusting VENC, it is possible to sensitize the sequence to slow or fast flows (see Q 7.13).

As commercially implemented by GE Medical Systems, PC MRA uses a four-point processing technique based on data acquired in an interleaved fashion throughout the sequence. These four components required to reconstruct the image include a GRE "mask" without flow encodings and three sets of paired data acquired when bipolar gradients are applied along the x, y and z axes. This complex data set is then combined into an image using either a phase subtraction or complex difference technique. The MR angiogram may be displayed as a magnitude flow image resembling that obtained from TOF techniques or as a phase map sensitive to flow direction.

In general, no uniform consensus exists as to which MRA technique is superior overall, although many authorities favor TOF methods for most applications. TOF sequences can be implemented on a wide range of scanners, and limits on field homogeneity are not as stringent for TOF sequences as for PC methods to obtain good-quality images. TOF sequences are most useful for imaging relatively rapid flow in vessels passing perpendicular to the plane of imaging (e.g., aorta, iliac, femoral, and carotid arteries). PC sequences appear to hold some advantage at present for imaging smaller and more tortuous vessels (e.g., distal branches of the middle cerebral artery) and large aneurysms with swirling flow. PC may also be superior to TOF techniques for MR venography. With each year, however, new advances in either type of sequence could significantly tip the balance one way or another, so the reader should keep abreast of developments in this field.

References

Dumoulin CL. Phase-contrast magnetic resonance angiography. Neuroimaging Clin North Am 2:657, 1992.

Keller PJ. Time-of-flight magnetic resonance angiography. Neuroimaging Clin North Am 2:639, 1992.

Q 7.13	What is VENC, and what happens if you choose it incorrectly?

VENC stands for velocity encoding, which is a parameter that must be specified by the operator to perform a PC MRA technique. VENC, measured in centimeters per second (cm/sec), should be chosen to encompass the highest velocities likely to be encountered within the vessel of interest. The VENC parameter adjusts the strength of the bipolar gradient so that the maximum velocity selected corresponds to a 180° phase shift in the data.

The VENC setting is critical for proper performance of the MRA pulse sequence but often can only be estimated since its optimum value is generally not known in advance. If VENC is chosen too high, the range of flows imaged will encompass only a limited number of degrees of phase

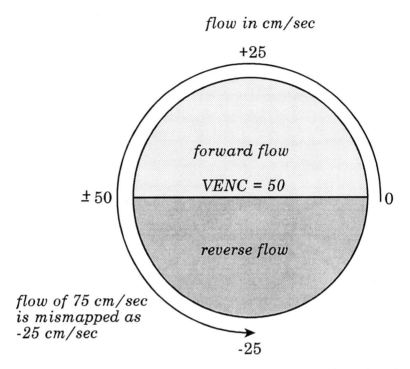

flow in cm/sec

Fig. 7-10. Velocity aliasing depends on the value of velocity encoding (VENC). With VENC of 50 cm/sec, a forward flow of 75 cm/sec cannot be distinguished from a reverse flow of 25 cm/sec.

shift. The signal-to-noise ratio (SNR) of the image is adversely affected, and vessels with slow flow may be difficult to see.

If VENC is picked too small, velocity aliasing may occur with faster flows not being appropriately represented. For example, if the chosen value of VENC is 50 cm/sec, the bipolar gradient is adjusted so that a flow of 25 cm/sec is assigned a phase of 90°, whereas a flow of 50 cm/sec is assigned 180° (Fig. 7-10). If the actual vessel velocity is 75 cm/sec, this flow is represented by a phase shift of 270°, which the computer cannot distinguish from a phase shift of −90°. Instead of representing the 75 cm/sec flow as its actual velocity, the computer will assign it a flow of 25 cm/sec in the opposite direction. Proper estimation of VENC is thus critical for successful PC MRA.

Reference

Turski P, Korosec F. Technical features and emerging clinical applications of phase-contrast magnetic resonance angiography. Neuroimaging Clin North Am 2:785, 1992.

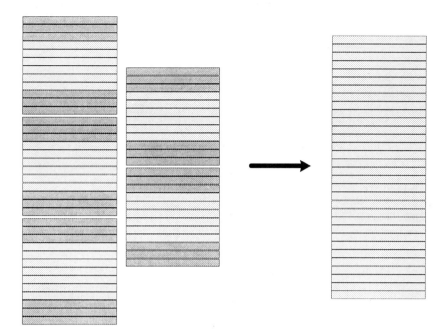

Fig. 7-11. MOTSA (multiple overlapping thin-slab acquisition). Darkly shaded slices are discarded in reconstruction of the final image.

Q	**What is MOTSA?**
7.14	

MOTSA, which stands for *m*ultiple *o*verlapping *t*hin-*s*lab *a*cquisition, is a hybrid between the 2DFT and 3DFT TOF techniques. MOTSA involves the acquisition of several thin (1.0 to 1.5 cm) overlapping 3DFT volumes. The use of narrow slabs minimizes troublesome saturation effects that reduce vessel signal in thick-slab 3DFT TOF imaging. Since contrast in the edge slices from these 3D slabs is suboptimal, MOTSA extracts only the central portions for each of the overlapping acquisitions to make up the final data set for processing into the MRA projections. This scheme is illustrated in Fig. 7-11.

References

Blatter DD, Parker DL, Robison RO. Cerebral MR angiography with multiple overlapping thin slab acquisition. Part I. Quantitative analysis of vessel visibility. Radiology 179:805, 1991.

Parker DL, Blatter DD. Multiple thin slab magnetic resonance angiography. Neuroimaging Clin North Am 2:677, 1992.

Q	**What is RACE?**
7.15	

RACE (*r*eal-time *a*cquisition and velocity *e*valuation) is a 1DFT method to extract velocity information from phase data. This technique does not produce an MR image but rather creates a time-velocity tracing similar to that seen on Doppler ultrasound through a vessel at a given point. RACE extracts this information by measuring the phase dispersions produced by the slice-selection gradient at various times throughout the cardiac cycle.

To acquire RACE data, a slice that is perpendicular to the direction of blood flow must first be selected by conventional MR imaging. Next, a narrow band within this plane is selected; this band should encompass the lumen of the vessel whose flow is to be measured. (This process is analogous to selecting a beam direction for a Doppler ultrasound measurement.) The RACE sequence itself is merely a short TR (~20 msec), short TE (~7 msec) GRE sequence that sequentially applies slice-select and read gradients perpendicular to the direction of flow but uses no phase-encode gradient. Because this fast sequence is acquired repeatedly throughout the cardiac cycle, it captures flow information with great temporal resolution. Since each data line is acquired in only 20 msec, flow information throughout the entire cardiac cycle is obtained without the need for cardiac gating by simply repeating the sequence many times.

The phase shifts measured are proportional to velocity of flow, but they also reflect motion contributions from everything within the projection (i.e., overlapping arteries, veins, and viscera). Even if these extraneous phase shifts could be removed by presaturation or projection dephasing, the velocity measured by RACE within a vessel still represents a spatially averaged velocity that may differ from Doppler measurements by as much as 33%. Nevertheless, RACE does offer a powerful new method for noninvasive blood flow measurements by MR and may prove useful in clinical practice as more experience is accumulated.

Reference

Haacke EM, Smith AS, Lin W et al. Velocity quantification in magnetic resonance imaging. Top Magn Reson Imaging 3:34, 1991.

| Q 7.16 | **What is VINNIE?** |

In contrast to RACE, VINNIE (velocity imaging in a cine mode) is a cardiac-gated 2D phase technique for measuring flow velocities. VINNIE data are acquired in a manner similar to that previously described for PC MRA, but VINNIE is more complex because data are acquired at multiple times throughout the cardiac cycle. This technique requires interleaving two scans where bipolar flow-encoding gradients are reversed relative to each other to generate phase changes in regions of flow. The resultant phase and magnitude data can be calibrated to provide measurements of flow velocity throughout the cardiac cycle. As in RACE, quantitative flow rates and even pressure gradients can be calculated by combining these velocity data with cross-sectional area measurements of the vessel. VINNIE provides spatial resolution of flows across the vessel that are not available in the 1D (RACE) method, but does so at the expense of increased imaging time.

Reference

Kondo C, Caputo GR, Semelka R et al. Right and left ventricular stroke volume measurements with velocity-encoded cine MR imaging: in vitro and in vivo validation. AJR 157:9, 1991.

| Q 7.17 | **What is the "dephase-rephase" technique?** |

This technique, or one of its variants, is an MRA method available on some systems (e.g., Siemens, Picker). In this technique, two data sets are acquired. In the first data set, flow signal is maximized by using gradient moment nulling; in the second set, flow signal is minimized by gradient-induced dephasing. Complex subtraction of the magnitude images from the two data sets produces an MR angiogram. Unfortunately, rephase-dephase methods have not proved particularly effective, being plagued by spatial misregistration artifacts, sensitivity to eddy currents and nonvascular motion, and limitations in dynamic range.

Reference

Doumoulin CL, Hart HR: MR angiography. Radiology 161:717, 1986.

Q
7.18

What is "black blood angiography?"

Black blood angiography is an alternative MRA strategy wherein the signal from flowing blood is suppressed (rendering it "black") rather than enhanced (as it is in most conventional MRA techniques). Rapidly flowing or turbulent blood has a naturally low signal because of phase dispersion and TOF signal losses. Suppression of signal from more slowly flowing blood is accomplished through the use of presaturation pulses and gradient-induced dephasing. Instead of a maximum intensity projection, a *minimum* intensity projection algorithm is used to generate the MR angiogram. Black blood angiography may have some usefulness for the imaging of certain vessels with rapid flow but has its own set of artifacts, including difficulties in distinguishing black blood from nearby vascular calcifications, cortical bone, and air.

Reference

Edelman RR, Mattle HP, Wallner B et al. Extracranial carotid arteries: evaluation with "black blood" MR angiography. Radiology 177:45, 1990.

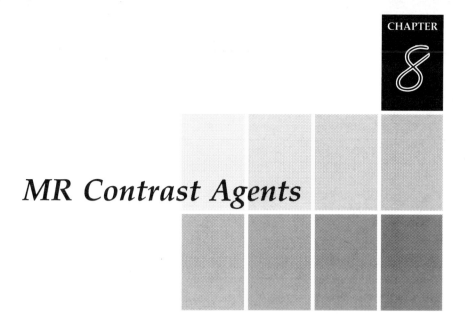

MR Contrast Agents

<table>
<tr><td>

Q

8.01
</td><td>

Why are most MR contrast agents based on the element gadolinium?
</td></tr>
</table>

Complexes of the element gadolinium (Gd) are the most widely used of currently available MR contrast agents. Gd is not directly seen in an MR image but manifests its presence indirectly by facilitating the relaxation of tissue hydrogen protons. These nearby protons interact not with the Gd nucleus, but rather with its electrons. Stated another way, the *electrons* of Gd interact with the resonating *protons* of hydrogen, allowing the protons to relax more rapidly.

Gd occupies the central position in the lanthanide series of elements. The lanthanide elements are grouped chemically because they possess partially filled inner shells of electrons (3d and 4f subshells). In its native state, Gd has seven unpaired electrons in its 4f orbitals, more than any other element. As with protons, electrons also have magnetic moments. Since the charge-to-mass ratio of the electron is much larger than that of the proton, however, the magnetic moment of an electron is also much greater than that of a proton. By virtue of its unique electronic structure, therefore, the Gd ion possesses a powerful magnetic moment. Furthermore, since the unpaired electrons producing this effect are located within inner shells, the powerful magnetic moment of Gd is largely maintained when the Gd ion is chelated to a ligand such as diethylenetriamine pentaacetic acid (DTPA).

Reference

Goldstein EJ, Burnett KR, Hansell JR et al. Gadolinium DTPA (an NMR proton imaging contrast agent): chemical structure, paramagnetic properties and pharmacokinetics. Physiol Chem Phys Med NMR 16:97, 1984.

Q 8.02	**Why does gadolinium apparently shorten only T1? Doesn't it have an effect on T2 as well?**

Because of its paramagnetic properties, Gd facilitates both longitudinal and transverse magnetic relaxation, thereby shortening *both* T1 and T2 of tissues in which it accumulates. The dominant effect (on T1 or T2) of such a contrast agent, however, depends on baseline tissue relaxation times in the absence of the agent, as well as the maximum tissue concentration achieved.

Theoretical analysis predicts that the relaxation rates observed after contrast administration $\{(1/T1)_{obs}$ and $(1/T2)_{obs}\}$ can be calculated as the sum of relaxation rates contributed by the native tissue and the paramagnetic agent, respectively:

$$(1/T1)_{obs} = (1/T1)_t + (1/T1)_p$$

$$(1/T2)_{obs} = (1/T2)_t + (1/T2)_p$$

where $(1/T1)_t$ and $(1/T2)_t$ are the relaxation rates of the tissue without contrast, and $(1/T1)_p$ and $(1/T2)_p$ are the relaxation rates attributable to the paramagnetic agent. Furthermore, $(1/T1)_p$ and $(1/T2)_p$ are linearly related to the concentration $[P]$ of the paramagnetic agent:

$$(1/T1)_p = R1\,[P]$$

$$(1/T2)_p = R2\,[P]$$

where $R1$ and $R2$ are called the "specific relaxivities" of the paramagnetic agent, measured in units of $(mmol/L \cdot sec)^{-1}$. Although this formulation is strictly true only for contrast agents dissolved in pure solvents and lacking solute-solute interactions, clinical measurements have demonstrated that it is nevertheless a reasonable approximation for the relaxation effects of Gd-DTPA in a variety of human tissues and tumors.

The relaxivities ($R1$ and $R2$) of Gd-DTPA are comparable; their measured values in aqueous solution are approximately 4 and 5 $(\text{mmol/L} \cdot \text{sec})^{-1}$, respectively. Because the $R1$ and $R2$ relaxivities are so similar, one might mistakenly conclude that Gd-DTPA would shorten $T1_{obs}$ and $T2_{obs}$ equally. This is not the case, however, because it is the relaxation *rates*, not relaxation *times*, that are additive and proportional to the concentration of Gd. Additionally, most biological tissues possess a marked natural disparity in their baseline relaxation times; $T1_t$ is often 5 to 10 times longer than $T2_t$ and therefore contributes further to the unequal effects of Gd on observed relaxation rates.

To demonstrate the apparent preferential T1 shortening effects of Gd at low doses, let us choose as our baseline tissue normal brain, in which $T1_t = 800$ msec (0.8 sec) and $T2_t = 80$ msec (0.08 sec). Let us now suppose the blood-brain barrier becomes disrupted, and Gd-DTPA accumulates in this tissue at a concentration of 0.1 mmol/L. According to the previous data and equations, the observed relaxation rates are

$$(1/T1)_{obs} = (1/.8) + (4)(.1) = 1.65 \text{ sec}^{-1}$$

$$(1/T2)^{obs} = (1/.08) + (5)(.1) = 13.0 \text{ sec}^{-1}$$

from which we calculate $T1_{obs} = 606$ msec and $T2_{obs} = 77$ msec. We can see that Gd has reduced the observed value of T1 by almost 25%, whereas it has diminished T2 by only 4%. In most tissues where T1 is normally much longer than T2, therefore, low concentrations of Gd-DTPA produce a relatively greater shortening of T1 than of T2.

Reference

Kirsch JE. Basic principles of magnetic resonance contrast agents. Top Magn Reson Imaging 3:1, 1991.

Q 8.03 **Can the T2-shortening effects of gadolinium ever be observed during routine spin echo (SE) imaging?**

In routine SE imaging the mild T2-shortening effects of low doses of Gd (which decrease signal intensity) are usually overwhelmed by the more dominant T1-shortening effects (which increase signal intensity) and are therefore not normally observed. However, as the concentration of Gd

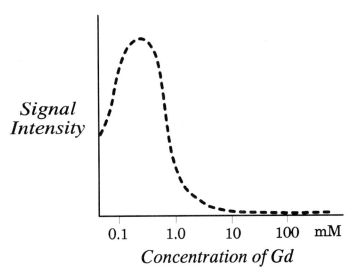

Fig. 8-1. Spin echo signal intensity as a function of gadolinium concentration [Gd]. MR signal intensity precipitously decreases once [Gd] passes a critical level.

increases, SE signal intensity eventually begins to fall (Fig. 8-1). The Gd concentration beyond which signal falls depends on the particular tissue and pulse sequence parameters selected.

Paradoxically decreased signal intensity of some tumors after contrast administration has been reported, but this is a rare phenomenon and is not normally encountered on routine SE images of most tissues using standard doses of Gd (0.1 to 0.3 mmol/kg). In the kidneys and bladder, however, where Gd is excreted and concentrated, tissue and urine levels of Gd may approach 40 mM. At concentrations this high, T2 shortening may result in a significant decrease in signal intensity noticeable on both T1-weighted and T2-weighted images. Urine in the bladder may exhibit an unusual triple-layering phenomenon (Fig. 8-2). T2-shortening effects predominate, and a low SE signal occurs in the bottom "pseudolayer" where Gd concentration is highest; in the middle layer, moderate concentrations of Gd result in T1 shortening and high SE signal.

Reference

Elster AD, Sobol WT, Hinson WH. Pseudolayering of Gd-DTPA in the urinary bladder. Radiology 174:379, 1990.

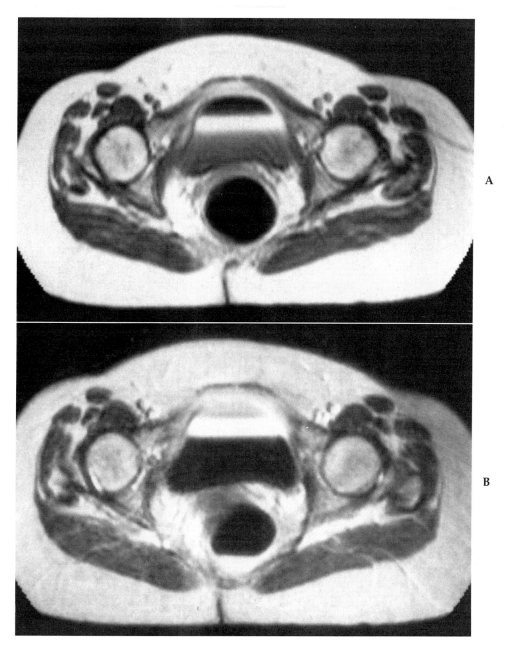

Fig. 8-2. "Pseudolayering" of Gd in the bladder. **A,** T1-weighted image. **B,** T2-weighted image. The top layer contains pure urine, whereas the middle and bottom pseudolayers contain increasing concentrations of Gd. T1-shortening effects predominate in the middle layer, resulting in increased signal intensity. T2-shortening effects predominate in the bottom layer, resulting in lower MR signal.

Q	Exactly how safe are the gadolinium-based MR contrast
8.04	agents?

Postmarketing surveillance studies of Gd-DTPA/dimeglumine (Magnevist) in Europe, Japan, and the United States have shown an extremely low incidence of adverse drug reactions. In a review of 13,439 patients, all the most common reactions were mild; they included nausea/vomiting (0.42%), local warmth/pain (0.41%), headache (0.26%), paresthesias (0.13%), and dizziness (0.10%). This reaction rate is comparable to that occurring during placebo injection of saline and is about one-third as common as reaction rates recorded with nonionic iodine-based contrast media.

Transient mild elevations of serum iron and bilirubin occur in approximately 30% and 3% of patients, respectively, who receive Gd-DTPA/dimeglumine. This dose-related effect is clinically inapparent. The mechanism by which Magnevist causes elevated iron and bilirubin levels is not known; possibilities include not only increased hemolysis, but also more rapid splenic clearance of older erythrocytes and alterations in the dynamics of iron transport. Elevations of iron and bilirubin apparently do not occur with gadoteridol (ProHance).

Moderately severe reactions, including bronchospasm, laryngospasm, facial edema, tachycardia, arrhythmias, or widespread urticaria, occur in about 1 in 5000 patients receiving Magnevist. Seizures induced directly by Magnevist in several epileptic patients have also been reported but are too rare to constitute evidence against the use of this drug to evaluate patients with seizures.

Worldwide, about a dozen severe anaphylactoid reactions to Magnevist have been reported. The incidence of such severe reactions is about 1 in 400,000 patients. Because of limited clinical experience to date, the relative safety of gadoteridol (ProHance) and gadodiamide (Omniscan) compared with Magnevist with regard to the incidence of severe reactions is unknown.

In conclusion, although the Gd-based MR contrast agents are extremely safe, they are not infinitely so. One should always remember that administration of any drug carries with it the risk of a life-threatening reaction.

Reference

Niendorf HP, Dinger JC, Haustein J et al. Tolerance data of Gd-DTPA: a review. Eur J Radiol 13:15, 1991.

Q
8.05

Has anyone actually died from them?

In mid-1992, Berlex/Schering reported details of two severe reactions to Magnevist, including one death. The details are as follows:

Case 1 (Virginia, December 1991). A 46-year-old woman with a history of asthma and bronchospasm was being evaluated by MR imaging for transient ischemic attacks to rule out cerebrovascular accident (stroke). The patient had been given aspirin prophylactically, even though she had related a history of aspirin allergy. During the unenhanced portion of the examination, she complained of itching and tingling. Immediately after administration of Magnevist, she became hypotensive, went into cardiopulmonary arrest, and could not be resuscitated.

Case 2 (Illinois, January 1992). A 44-year-old man was undergoing spinal MR imaging to diagnose suspected recurrent disk herniation. He had a long history of bronchopulmonary disease (asthma, bronchitis, emphysema) and was dependent on inhalant bronchodilators and steroids. Immediately after administration of Magnevist, the patient uttered, "I'm having an asthma attack!" The medical staff in the MR suite immediately administered the patient his inhalant bronchodilator without relief. Progressive laryngospasm and bronchospasm made intubation difficult, and only after multiple attempts was an airway established. The patient suffered severe anoxic brain injury and remains in a comatose state at a full-care facility.

As a result of these two severe reactions, Berlex added a warning to its most recent package insert to include cautious use of the agent in patients with a history of asthma or other allergic respiratory disorders. Since that time, one additional death has been reported in an elderly woman with no history of asthma.

Reference

Safety and efficacy of Magnevist (gadopentetate dimeglumine) injection: four years of experience. April 1992. (Available from Medical Affairs, Berlex Laboratories, tel 201-292-3007.)

Q
8.06

With the possibility, even remote, of a severe reaction to gadolinium, should a physician or other health care provider skilled in advanced cardiac life support and resuscitation equipment always be present on site when it is administered?

In my opinion, the answer is "yes." Although extremely rare, such life-threatening reactions can and do occur, and appropriate staff and equipment should be immediately available to handle such emergencies. Although the risk of a severe reaction to Gd is extremely small, it is not zero. Although Gd agents are much safer than iodine agents, the same standards of care should be applied to both.

(This opinion was also shared by the consensus panel on MR contrast agents at the 1992 RSNA scientific assembly.)

Q 8.07

The labeling information for Magnevist contains an apparent paradox concerning the drug's pharmacokinetics. On one hand, the mean elimination half-life is reported to be 1.6 hours, yet only 91% of the drug is said to be excreted within 24 hours. With a half-life this short, shouldn't 99.99% be excreted in this period?

Perceptive questions such as this keep me in academics. When this paradox was first proposed to me by an astute resident last year, I had no answer. To my knowledge, this issue has never been addressed in any of the pharmacokinetic studies of Gd-DTPA reported in the literature. The answer is known but is buried among internal and Food and Drug Administration (FDA) documents from phase I and II clinical trials at Berlex/Schering.

Conventional kinetic analyses show that over the first 6 hours after intravenous injection of Gd-DTPA, the concentrations of the drug in plasma decline according to a biexponential function, which can be explained by a distribution phase with a mean half-life of 0.20 ± 0.13 hours and a disposition/elimination phase with a half-life of 1.58 ± 0.13 hours. Notwithstanding, approximately 9% of the administered dose remains in the body at 24 hours and is excreted gradually through the urine and feces during the next week. Therefore, about 10% of an administered dose of Gd-DTPA becomes sequestered in some compartment, presumably in the extracellular interstitium, and does not freely exchange bidirectionally with the plasma. The freely exchangeable Gd-DTPA, representing 90% of the total, is completely excreted over 24 hours. The sequestered form, however, representing 10% of the total, is slowly released and excreted over several days' time.

Reference

Weinmann HJ, Laniado M, Mützel W. Pharmacokinetics of GdDTPA/dimeglumine after intravenous injection into healthy volunteers. Physiol Chem Physics Med NMR 16:167, 1984.

Q   **Can gadolinium be given safely to infants and children?**

All available evidence suggests that Gd-DTPA is well tolerated in infants and children and may provide useful radiological information in selected cases. The risk of an adverse drug reaction is apparently no higher or lower in the pediatric population than in adults. At least three severe hypotensive reactions to Magnevist in children have now been reported, although none has resulted in permanent injury.

Since newborns and young infants have significantly lower glomerular filtration and renal clearance rates than do older children and adults, the biological half-life of Gd-based MR contrast agents is prolonged. In a full-term newborn the half-life is 6.5 hours; it may be longer than 9 hours in premature infants. By 2 months of age, the adult value of 1.5 hours is attained.

This prolonged half-life in newborns and young infants results in persisting enhancement of normal structures for up to several hours after injection (Fig. 8-3). The prolonged half-life thus provides an increased window of time for performing imaging in these patients. For example, a sedated infant who awakes during contrast infusion may be removed from the imager, resedated, and reimaged within 1 to 2 hours without the need for injection of additional Gd-DTPA. Alternatively, if only a postcontrast study is desired, the infant may be sedated and given the contrast infusion while still in the neonatal care unit and then may undergo nonurgent MR imaging.

References

Elster AD. Cranial MR imaging with Gd-DTPA in neonates and young infants: preliminary experience. Radiology 176:225, 1990.

Elster AD, Rieser GD. Gd-DTPA-enhanced cranial MR imaging in children: initial clinical experience and recommendation for its use. AJNR 10:1027, 1989.

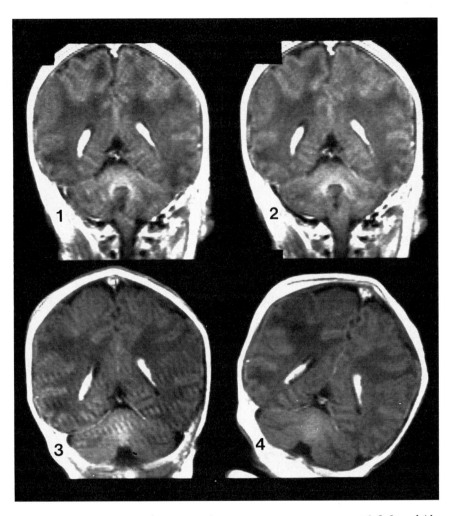

Fig. 8-3. Persistent contrast enhancement in a premature neonate seen at 1, 2, 3, and 4 hours after Gd injection. The prolonged half-life (4 to 9 hours) of Gd in neonates and young infants provides an expanded window of opportunity for performing postcontrast imaging.

Q 8.09	If neonates and young infants have lower renal excretion rates of MR contrast agents than adults do, should they receive a lower dose?

Although renal excretion of Gd-based contrast agents is prolonged in neonates and young infants, other factors must be considered in determining the optimum dose to be administered for imaging. Renal excretion rates aside, neonates have twice the volume of extracellular fluid that adults have in proportion to their body weights. Therefore, neonates and young infants who receive Gd-DTPA on a dose-per-kilogram basis have blood Gd-DTPA concentrations only one-half those in adults after equilibration. This fact argues against using a lower dose per kilogram in infants than in adults, even though the serum half-life is prolonged. Clinical experience by our group and others has demonstrated that the adult dose of Gd-DTPA (0.1 mmol/kg) is also appropriate in infants and children.

Reference

Elster AD. Cranial MR imaging with Gd-DTPA in neonates and young infants: preliminary experience. Radiology 176:225, 1990.

| Q | Can gadolinium-based contrast agents be used safely in |
| 8.10 | patients with renal failure or insufficiency? |

Although the FDA labeling for Magnevist indicates caution in its use in patients with renal failure or insufficiency, administration of most Gd-based contrast agents is nevertheless probably safe in these clinical circumstances. Several dozen patients with moderately severe chronic renal failure have been studied after administration of either Gd-DTPA or gadoterate meglumine (Gd-DOTA), and no significant or permanent adverse effects on renal function have been noted. However, a few patients receiving Gd-DOTA have had their serum creatinine levels transiently increase by 10% to 25%, and some receiving Gd-DTPA have temporarily shown mildly elevated excretion of urinary β-NAG, a sensitive indicator of proximal renal tubule cell injury. Renal tolerance of nonionic Gd agents is unknown, but we might even expect them to be safer than Gd-DTPA or Gd-DOTA, paralleling the experience with iodinated contrast agents.

The biological half-life of MR contrast agents is prolonged in patients with renal failure or insufficiency, as is true of other drugs that are excreted principally by glomerular filtration. A single hemodialysis treatment removes about 75% of the administered dose.

On the basis of this data, I do not hesitate to give MR contrast to patients with renal failure or insufficiency if I believe the presence (or absence) of contrast enhancement will add significantly to my diagnostic accuracy in a particular situation. Because of potential systemic toxicity effects of the free Gd ion, however, I do recommend that patients who require hemodialysis be dialyzed within 24 hours after Gd administration, if possible. Additionally, I prefer to administer gadoteriol (ProHance) in this situation, since its dissociation constant is slightly higher than that of either Magnevist or Omniscan and in theory should be less likely to release free Gd if retained in the body for a prolonged time. It should also be recognized that, as with iodine contrast, several dialyses may be necessary to remove the agent completely.

References

Bellin M-F, Deray G, Assogba U et al. Gd-DOTA: evaluation of its renal tolerance in patients with chronic renal failure. Magn Reson Imaging 10:115, 1992.

Haustein J, Niendorf PH, Krestin G et al. Renal tolerance of gadolinium-DTPA/dimeglumine in patients with chronic renal failure. Invest Radiol 27:153, 1992.

| Q |
| 8.11 |

What are the principal differences among the several gadolinium-based contrast agents that are now being marketed?

Four Gd-based contrast agents for intravenous administration are now being used and tested nationally or internationally (Table 8-1). Two of these are ionic (Magnevist, Dotarem) and two are nonionic (Omniscan, ProHance). Dotarem is being marketed in Europe, but I understand Guerbet/Schering has no plans to introduce this agent into the U.S. market. The other three agents are currently FDA approved and being actively marketed both in North America and elsewhere. The chemical structures of these four Gd chelates are presented schematically in Fig. 8-4.

Gd-DTPA (Magnevist) is a linear ionic complex based around the chelate diethylenetriamine pentaacetic acid (DTPA). The Gd^{+3} ion bonds with three of DTPA's carboxyl (CO_2^-) groups, forming a (−2)-charged complex known as *gadopentetate*. In its formulation as Magnevist, each mole of the (gadopentetate)$^{-2}$ moiety is ionically balanced with two moles of (meglumine)$^{+1}$, resulting in the compound *gadopentetate dimeglumine*. Since three osmotically active components are associated with each atom of Gd administered, the osmolality of this agent is relatively high (1940 mOsm/L).

| TABLE | 8-1. Gadolinium-Based MR Contrast Agents |

Trade Name	Chemical Name	Company	Type	Osmolality (mOsm/kg)
Magnevist	Gd-DTPA, gadopentetate dimeglumine	Berlex/Schering	Ionic	1960
Dotarem	Gd-DOTA, gadoterate meglumine	Guerbet/ Schering	Ionic	1170
Omniscan	Gd-DTPA-BMA, gadodiamide	Sanofi/ Winthrop	Nonionic	789
ProHance	Gd-HP-D03A, gadoteridol	Squibb	Nonionic	630

Gadodiamide (Omniscan) is a linear nonionic complex based around the backbone DTPA-BMA (bismethylamide). In this molecule, two of the DTPA carboxyl groups have been replaced by $CO-NHCH_3$, resulting in a (–3)-charged chelate that is exactly balanced by the Gd^{+3} ion, making the agent nonionic and allowing its pharmaceutical osmolality to be low (789 mOsm/L). However, because of the loss of the two extra carboxyl groups, the affinity of the chelate for the Gd ion is reduced, resulting in somewhat higher levels of free Gd in this drug than the others.

Gd-DOTA (Dotarem) is based on the macrocyclic chelate tertraazacyclo-dodecane tetraacetic acid (DOTA). The macrocyclic formulation results in an affinity constant of the ligand for Gd several orders of magnitude larger than gadopentetate or gadodiamide. Because the Gd-DOTA complex has a –1 charge, a counterbalancing cation is necessary to obtain zero net charge; thus, Dotarem is an ionic agent with two osmotically active particles per atom of Gd, with a formulation osmolality of 1170 mOsm/L.

Gadoteridol (ProHance) is based on a macrocyclic ligand similar to DOTA, except one of the carboxyl groups has been replaced by $CH(OH)CH_3$. This replacement confers on the ligand a –3 charge, which exactly balances the Gd^{+3} ion, resulting in a nonionic complex with low osmolality and excellent in vitro stability.

Reference

Tweedle MF, Eaton SM, Eckelman WC et al. Comparative chemical structure and pharmacokinetics of MRI contrast agents. Invest Radiol 23(suppl 1):S236, 1988.

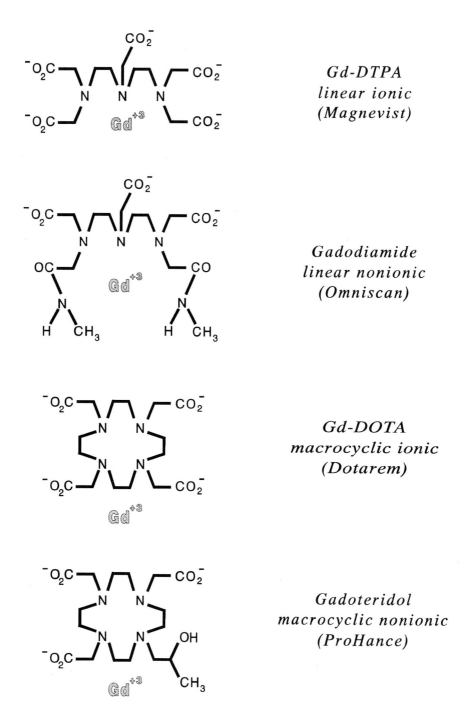

Fig. 8-4. Structures of the principal Gd-based contrast agents now commercially available. (See Q 8.11 for details.)

Q
8.12

But are the new agents really any safer or better?

Preliminary data from the clinical trials of these new agents suggest that their safety profiles are similar to that of Magnevist. It should be realized, however, that large-scale postmarketing surveillance studies have not yet been performed, and therefore statistically accurate comparisons among these agents are not possible.

Naturally, drug salespeople for the new Gd agents attempt to draw parallels with the advantages and greater safety of nonionic *iodine* agents. Although this analogy is appealing, it is not entirely accurate. One must recall that the osmolar toxicity of a contrast agent is determined not by its concentration in the bottle, but by its concentration in the blood. The blood concentration of a contrast agent depends on its total osmotic load, which is the drug's pharmaceutical osmolality times the volume administered.

For example, the total osmolar load from a 15 ml dose of Magnevist is approximately 35 mOsm, whereas the osmolar load from the same dose of ProHance would be only 9 mOsm. (For comparison, serum plasma has an osmolality of about 285 mOsm/L.) Administration of either of these drugs would increase serum osmolality by less than 5%. Iodinated agents, however, are administered in much larger doses, so that their osmolar effects are much greater. For example, the total osmolar load from 150 ml of Renograffin-60 (osmolarity, 1420 mOsm/L) is calculated to be 213 mOsm, whereas the osmolar load from 150 ml of Isovue-300 (osmolality, 616 mOsm/kg) is 122 mOsm. Clearly, therefore, *ionic* Gd agents result in a lower serum osmotic load than even *nonionic* iodine agents. The difference between ionic and nonionic Gd agents in terms of their osmotic effect is therefore not nearly as great as that between ionic and nonionic iodine agents.

The amount of free Gd in each formulation is an issue in theory, with ProHance having the least and Omniscan having the most free Gd of all the agents listed. In the dosages administered, however, there is no evidence that the small differences in free Gd among these various formulations is of any clinical significance.

Q
8.13

In which patients should MR contrast agents be routinely administered?

In cranial MR imaging, we generally decide which patients will receive contrast material before the scan on the basis of clinical and historical factors that have proved to be "high yield": lesion seen on previous computed tomography (CT) or noncontrast MR studies, prior surgery for intracranial tumor, history of cardiovascular disease, history of extracranial malignancy, advancing patient age, sepsis/infection, and objective neurological deficits. Low-yield factors include nonspecific complaints (e.g., headache, dizziness), epilepsy, and age less than 35 years.

In the extracranial head and neck, we use contrast primarily to characterize lesions of the orbit and to evaluate the spread of tumors arising in the nasopharynx and skull base.

In spinal imaging, we use Gd only in the following circumstances: to distinguish scar from epidural fibrosis, to characterize the cause of a syrinx or cord enlargement, and in patients with suspected metastatic disease.

In body imaging, MR contrast may be useful to differentiate benign from malignant breast masses, to identify regions of myocardial ischemia, and to characterize certain liver and adrenal masses. Dynamic contrast-enhanced imaging may be useful in evaluation of certain medical renal diseases and in renal transplant recipients.

The full extent of musculoskeletal tumors and infections may be better characterized through the use of Gd combined with fat suppression techniques.

References

Bydder GM. Clinical applications of contrast agents in body imaging. Top Magn Reson Imaging 3:74, 1991.

Elster AD, Moody DM, Ball MR, Laster DW. Is Gd-DTPA required for routine cranial MR imaging? Radiology 173:231, 1989.

Q   **Is there any role for high-dose or half-dose regimens?**

The usefulness of double-dose and triple-dose regimens in patients with suspected cerebral metastatic disease has been documented in the phase III clinical trials of ProHance. In a number of anecdotal examples, these high-dose protocols demonstrated more cerebral metastases than were seen with the standard (0.1 mmol/kg) dose. Although the difference between nine metastases and 10 metastases is not clinically significant, the distinction between zero and one or between one and two may be critical for proper diagnosis and management. Further studies are therefore needed to determine the true benefit and potential limitations in these high-dose regimens.

Some interest has been devoted to half-dose regimens, mainly from the standpoint of cost containment. However, the data from the ProHance trials seem to support the concept that more, rather than less, is better. An exception may be found in the evaluation of pituitary disease, where a half dose has been shown to be just as effective as a full dose. Here, too much enhancement of normal pituitary tissue may actually impede the diagnosis of microadenomas.

References

Davis PC, Gokhale KA, Joseph GJ et al. Pituitary adenoma: correlation of half-dose gadolinium-enhanced MR imaging with surgical findings in 26 patients. Radiology 180:779, 1991.

Yuh WTC, Engelken JD, Muhonen MG et al. Experience with high dose gadolinium MR imaging in the evaluation of brain metastases. AJNR 13:335, 1992.

Q **Can gadolinium contrast be given to pregnant or lactating women?**

Gd-DTPA has been shown to cross the placenta and even appear in the fetal bladder during MR imaging. Because the effects of this drug on the developing fetus are largely unknown, I administer Gd-DTPA to pregnant women only in exceptional circumstances where the potential diagnostic benefits appear paramount.

Gd-DTPA has also been shown to be excreted in breast milk, but only a tiny fraction of the administered dose can be detected after 24 hours. I therefore recommend that breast-feeding be suspended for 24 hours after administration of Gd-DTPA.

Reference

Rofsky NM, Weinreb JC, Litt AW. Quantitative analysis of gadopentate dimeglumine excreted in breast milk. JMRI 3:131, 1993.

Q **What types of bowel MR contrast agents are available?**

A wide range of both water-soluble and immiscible materials that either increase or decrease the signal intensity of the intestinal lumen are currently in various stages of testing and development. Dilute solutions of Geritol (ferric ammonium citrate) are FDA approved and have long been used in many centers as a gastrointestinal contrast agent for MR imaging. This regimen, although quite successful for opacifying the stomach and duodenum, becomes increasingly unreliable beyond the proximal jejunum as a result of dilution and mixing effects.

One promising current strategy involves the oral administration of a 10 ml/kg formulation of 1.0 mM Gd-DTPA in solution with 15 g mannitol/L. In clinical trials in Europe, this regimen successfully marked the distal small bowel within 90 minutes of administration.

Reference

Laniado M, Kornmesser W, Hamm B et al. MR imaging of the gastrointestinal tract: value of Gd-DTPA. AJR 150:817, 1988.

Q 8.17	**What is the current status of ferrites and the other liver agents?**

Particulate agents such as ferrites and superparamagnetic iron oxide crystals have excited considerable interest as possible MR contrast media for liver and reticuloendothelial system imaging. Unlike water-soluble MR contrast agents (e.g., Gd-DTPA), particulate agents have larger physical size and correspondingly greater magnetic moments because of molecular exchange coupling and the formation of magnetic domains. Although both T1 and T2 are shortened, the dominant effect is on T2. The apparent mechanism of this preferential T2 shortening by these large particles results from their bulk susceptibility effects; that is, they cause a significant local distortion of the nearby magnetic fields. Water molecules diffusing near these particles become dephased from the local inhomogeneities, and T2 signal loss ensues.

Ferrites and superparamagnetic iron particles are phagocytized by the Kupffer cells lining the hepatic sinusoids and are not deposited in neoplastic mass lesions such as metastases. Because of their predominant T2-shortening effects, they cause normal liver to have low signal on MR images and highlight abnormal tissue sharply.

FDA approval for the human trials of these agents has moved slowly, however, because of several severe hypotensive reactions encountered in one company's formulation. Theoretical concerns have also been expressed about potential hepatic toxicity from iron overload and the unknown long-term effects of persistent nondegraded particles remaining in the reticuloendothelial system. (Remember Thorotrast?) Considering these problems, I would not expect the iron particulates to be commercially available before 1995.

A hepatic agent that may receive earlier approval than ferrites is manganese dipyridoxal diphosphate (Mn-DPDP). This enzymatically active analog of vitamin B_6 is taken up selectively by hepatocytes. As with Gd-DTPA, its primary effect is to shorten T1. Normal liver tissue is therefore enhanced on T1-weighted images, and non-hepatocyte-containing masses appear dark.

References

Elizondo G, Fretz CJ, Stark DD et al. Preclinical evaluation of Mn-DPDP: a new paramagnetic hepatobiliary agent for MR imaging. Radiology 178:73, 1991.

Stark DD, Weissleder R, Elizondo G et al. Superparamagnetic iron oxide: clinical application as a contrast agent for MR imaging of the liver. Radiology 168:287, 1988.

Advanced MR Imaging Techniques

This chapter focuses on several advanced MR techniques that have only recently been widely introduced to clinical sites and some even newer techniques that will soon become available. Also described are several promising avenues of research in MR that are likely to become clinically useful and commercially available during the next several years.

Q

9.01

What is magnetization transfer imaging?

Magnetization transfer (MT) imaging is a new technique in which image contrast is modulated by selectively saturating a pool of protons in macromolecules and their associated "bound" water. The usual version of the method involves applying a presaturation pulse with a bandwidth of a few hundred hertz and center frequency shifted from the water resonance by 1000 to 2500 Hz, followed by gradient spoiling to avoid interference patterns with the next radiofrequency (RF) pulse. This off-resonance pulse has sufficient power to saturate protons in the immobile pool without directly affecting those in free water (Fig. 9-1). After the MT saturation pulse, a routine imaging sequence is performed. By saturating the bound proton pool, new tissue relaxation characteristics and image contrasts may be revealed.

As discussed in Q 2.15, dipolar cross-relaxation between free water protons and protons on macromolecules is an important determinant of T1 and T2 in many tissues, especially those with a high protein content, such

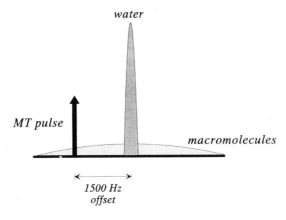

Fig. 9-1. Magnetization transfer (MT) pulse applied far off water resonance saturates the broad macromolecular pool of hydrogen with short T2 values. Because bound water interacts closely with this pool, some saturation of the water peak indirectly occurs through dipolar interactions.

as liver and brain. MT pulses are believed to act by saturating protons in this macromolecular reservoir as well as the associated and closely coupled water protons in their hydration spheres. After an MT pulse is applied, the MR signal is reduced for tissues in which macromolecular-water interactions are an important mechanism of relaxation.

This suppression of background tissue by MT pulses makes the technique a useful adjunct to MR angiography (MRA). Preliminary studies have shown small vessel detail and contrast are significantly improved in time of flight (TOF) MRA when MT pulses are employed.

A second potential use of MT pulses is in conjunction with contrast-enhanced T1-weighted images. Because gadolinium (Gd) enhancement is caused by a water–Gd ion interaction (not macromolecular cross-relaxation), MT pulses suppress the signal from background tissues and render Gd-enhanced areas more conspicuous.

A third potential use of MT pulses is in conjunction with T2-weighted images when early demyelination or protein destruction may be detected before its appearance on routine images. In this application, diseased tissues with altered protein-water interactions are less suppressed by the MT pulses, rendering them more conspicuous on T2-weighted images.

The amount of MT can be quantitated by obtaining two sets of images (one with an MT pulse and one without it) and then digitally subtracting them. The magnetization transfer ratio (MTR) may be defined as

$$MTR = \frac{M_o - M_s}{M_o}$$

where M_o is the magnitude of tissue signal before the MT pulse, and M_s is the signal when the pulse is on.

Despite these apparent advantages, MT imaging techniques are beset with certain inherent problems and limitations. First, MT pulses are not slice selective, require high RF power, and deposit significant energy in the tissue, which may result in exceeding specific absorption rate (SAR) limits. Second, MTR measurements are not specific, are susceptible to motion-related errors, and vary significantly as a function of the shape, bandwidth, and frequency offset of the MT pulse. Finally, the signal from fat is not appreciably affected by MT pulses, since storage lipids are chemically and physically isolated from the bulk water reservoir in most tissues. Therefore, *both* fat suppression and MT pulses may be necessary to improve angiographic or Gd contrast in fat-containing organs and tissues.

References

Elster AD, King JC, Mathews VM, Hamilton C. Improved detection of gadolinium enhancement using magnetization transfer imaging. Neuroimaging Clin North Am 1993 (in press).

Wolff SD, Balaban RS. Magnetization transfer contrast (MTC) and tissue water proton relaxation in vivo. Magn Reson Med 10:135, 1989.

| Q 9.02 | How is fat suppression accomplished? |

In clinical MR imaging and spectroscopy, several different techniques have been employed to reduce (suppress) the signal from fat. These methods can be broadly classified as (1) phase evolution (Dixon and Chopper pulse methods), (2) frequency-selective excitation/saturation ("fat sat," CHESS), (3) T1-dependent suppression (STIR), and (4) miscellaneous (selective water excitation, slice-selective gradient reversal). These techniques are described in more detail in Q 9.03 to Q 9.06.

| Q 9.03 | What is the "phase evolution" method of fat suppression? |

As discussed in Q 6.04, fat and water protons resonate at slightly different frequencies by virtue of the 3.5 parts per million (ppm) chemical shift

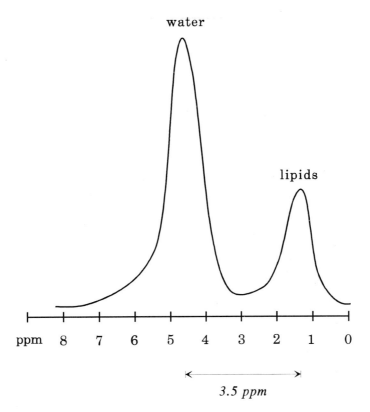

Fig. 9-2. Typical fat and water spectra on a clinical imager have peaks differing by about 3.5 ppm.

between them (Fig. 9-2). At 1.5 T, fat and water protons fall alternately in and out of phase with each other every 2.2 msec (see Fig. 6-4). Phase evolution methods use these time-dependent phase shifts between water and fat to suppress the fat (or water) signals selectively.

In 1984 Dixon proposed a chemical shift imaging method in which two sets of images were acquired: one routine spin echo (SE) image with fat and water signals in phase and another with the timing of the 180° pulse adjusted by a few milliseconds so that the fat and water signals were out of phase at the center of the echo. The signal intensities of the two images (I_1 and I_2) obtained with the Dixon method can be written

$$I_1 = W + F \text{ and } I_2 = W - F$$

where W and F are the signal contributions from water and fat, respectively. By image addition or subtraction ($I_1 + I_2 = 2W$; $I_1 - I_2 = 2F$), pure "water" and "fat" images can then be reconstructed.

Numerous modifications of the Dixon method have been subsequently proposed, including the Chopper method (incorporating phase alternation of the RF) and gradient echo (GRE) implementations. Today, however, most of these phase contrast fat suppression methods have been largely supplanted by frequency-selective techniques (discussed next).

Reference

Dixon WT. Simple proton spectroscopic imaging. Radiology 153:189, 1984.

Q 9.04	How do "fat sat" pulses work?

Because the resonance frequencies of water and fat are separated by about 3.5 ppm, it is possible to saturate selectively the spectral peak of either water or fat using a narrow-bandwidth, frequency-selective RF ("fat sat") pulse before imaging (Fig. 9-3, *A*). Several variations of this method are possible.

In "true" *saturation* methods, a several-hundred-millisecond, low-intensity RF pulse is applied after careful center frequency calibration of the fat resonance has been performed (see Q 3.17). This long-duration saturation pulse rotates the fat magnetization many times around the direction of the applied RF field. In conjunction with simultaneous T1 and T2 relaxation, the *z* component of fat magnetization is driven to zero (nulled). After complete saturation of the fat resonance has been attained, the unexcited water component can then be imaged using a conventional pulse sequence. Although true saturation methods are frequently employed in spectroscopy, they are not routinely used in clinical MR imaging because of their concomitant high RF power deposition and increase in imaging time.

In modern clinical MR imaging, fat suppression is generally accomplished by means of a "homospoil" technique, usually some variation of a method known as CHESS (*Chemical Shift Selection*). In this method a short-duration, frequency-selective 90° RF pulse is first applied that rotates the fat magnetization into the transverse plane (Fig. 9-3, *B*). While in the transverse plane, the fat magnetization is dephased by application of a spoiler gradient. This process theoretically leaves only the magnetization of water aligned with the *z* axis and available to participate in the ensuing pulse sequence.

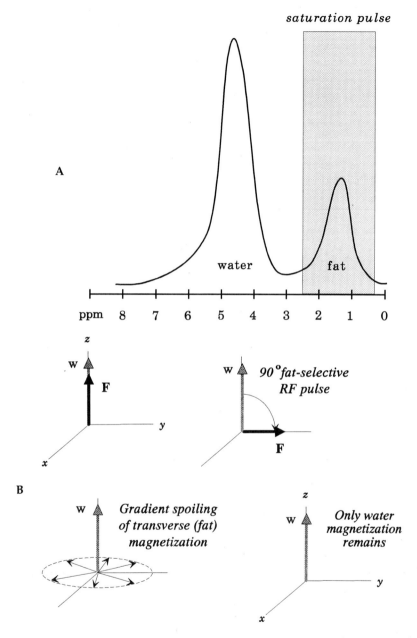

Fig. 9-3. **A,** The fat (or water) peak may be selectively saturated by a narrow-bandwidth radiofrequency (RF) pulse. **B,** "Fat sat" pulses on most commercial imagers are variations of the CHESS method pictured here. (See Q 9.04 for details.)

On most MR imagers the "fat sat" pulse is gaussian shaped or sinc shaped with a bandwidth of about 200 Hz and a pulse length of 10 to 15 msec. For spectroscopic applications, more complex pulse trains may be used. These variations include binomial, multinomial (e.g., "1331"), and self-refocusing pulses.

Frequency-selective fat suppression techniques are useful principally on high-field scanners where magnetic field homogeneity is excellent. Even on these highly homogeneous scanners, suppression of fat signal may be nonuniform, particularly when the field of view (FOV) is large. On scanners in which the magnetic field varies across the FOV by more than 3.5 ppm, frequency-selective techniques cannot be employed. On these systems another method (usually STIR, see Q 9.05) must be used to achieve fat suppression.

Reference

Keller PJ, Hunter WW Jr, Schmalbrock P. Multisection fat-water imaging with chemical shift selective presaturation. Radiology 164:539, 1987.

Q 9.05 **What is STIR?**

STIR stands for short TI inversion recovery (TI, inversion time) and is a popular technique for fat suppression that is applicable at all field strengths. In a standard inversion recovery sequence the longitudinal magnetization is first inverted by a 180° pulse, followed by a time delay (TI) of 100 to several hundred milliseconds. During this time delay, regrowth of longitudinal magnetization occurs before a signal is generated. The regrowth of longitudinal magnetization is dictated by the T1 (distinguish from TI) of the tissues being imaged. Fat, with very short T1 values (250 to 350 msec), has a rapid regrowth of its longitudinal magnetization. In most other tissues, with inherently longer T1 values, regrowth of the longitudinal magnetization is less rapid. This principle is illustrated in Fig. 9-4. The point at which each tissue crosses through zero is called its *null point*.

Since the longitudinal magnetization $M_L(t)$ at a time after the inversion pulse is a simple exponential returning to equilibrium value M_o with time constant T1, we can write

$$M_L(t) = M_o(1 - 2e^{-t/T1})$$

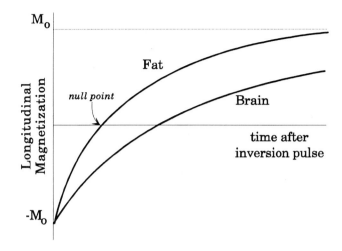

Fig. 9-4. Longitudinal magnetization in the STIR sequence. The inversion time (TI) is adjusted to null the signal from fat.

From this equation we can easily see that $M_L(t) = 0$ when $e^{-t/T1} = \frac{1}{2}$, or $t = (ln\ 2)\ T1 \approx 0.69\ T1$. Since the T1 of fat is about 250 msec, its null point will occur when $t = TI = 170$ to 180 msec. An inversion recovery sequence with such a short TI value is known as a STIR sequence.

With the shortest T1 of most naturally occurring substances in the body, fat passes through its null point before other tissues do. At the time of signal formation in the STIR sequence, therefore, nearly all other tissues have negative values of longitudinal magnetization. However, since a magnitude image is reconstructed from these data, these negative values are inverted and appear bright in the final image in direct proportion to their T1 values. Thus the STIR sequence has one additional useful feature besides fat suppression: it produces tissue contrast wherein tissues with long T1 values (e.g., cerebrospinal fluid, tumors) appear bright. This effect is directly opposite to contrast obtained in SE pulse sequences, in which long T1 values reduce the signal. In STIR sequences, therefore, T1 and T2 effects are additive, whereas they are competitive in conventional SE imaging.

In clinical practice, the STIR technique is useful for fat suppression on low-field and inhomogeneous magnets with which frequency-selective saturation (see Q 9.04) cannot be performed. STIR is particularly useful in the orbit to suppress fat and highlight lesions of the optic nerve (Fig. 9-5). It is also valuable in bone marrow imaging, in which normal marrow fat is effectively suppressed and metastatic lesions are rendered more conspicuous.

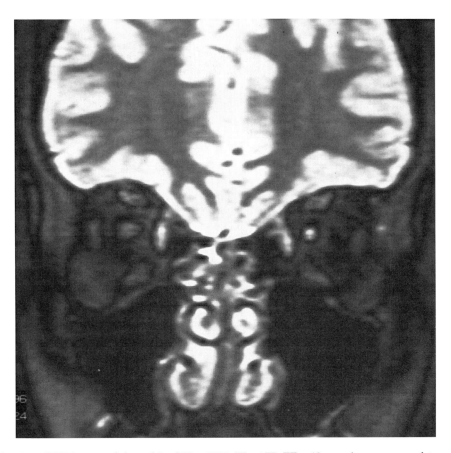

Fig. 9-5. STIR image of the orbits (TR = 1500, TI = 175, TE = 40 msec) suppresses fat well and demonstrates brain contrast that is proportional to additive T1 and T2 values.

Reference

Elster AD. Cranial magnetic resonance imaging. New York: Churchill Livingstone, 1988, p 25.

Q 9.06	What other fat suppression methods are available?

Several other fat suppression methods have been experimentally investigated but have yet to attain widespread commercial implementation. These include spectroscopic techniques, water-selective excitation (3D-FATS), and hybrid methods. One unique fat suppression method, *slice-selective gradient reversal,* deserves special mention because it is used as the principal method of fat suppression on MR scanners manufactured by Picker. In this clever technique, an accentuated chemical shift misregistration in the slice-select direction is first induced by using a narrow-bandwidth 90° RF pulse in conjunction with a reduced strength of slice-select gradient. The slice-select gradient is then activated with reversed polarity at the time of the 180° pulse. Because fat protons are shifted out of the slice in different directions between the 90° and 180° pulses, only water protons are stimulated by *both* the 90° and 180° pulses. Fat protons are chemically shifted so that they receive either the 90° or 180° pulse, but not both. Picker users should be familiar with this method, whose details can be found in the reference cited next.

Reference

Axel L, Glover G, Pelc N. Chemical-shift magnetic resonance imaging of two-line spectra by gradient reversal. Magn Reson Med 2:428, 1985.

Q 9.07	How does one obtain spectra instead of images on an MR scanner?

In conventional MR imaging, we obtain signals emitted by hydrogen nuclei from small voxels that have been selected by spatial variations in frequency and phase. By using frequency changes for spatial encoding, however, we have lost our ability to discriminate much of the important information about chemical shifts among the nuclei. The signals from water, fat, and other hydrogen-containing molecules all combine to produce a single net signal from each voxel, and in general, we have little ability to distinguish the relative contributions of each. Magnetic resonance spectroscopy (MRS) seeks to extract this chemical shift information in both a qualitative and a quantitative manner. Additionally, MRS techniques probe the signals and chemical shift information from other nuclei of potential physiological interest (e.g., ^{31}P, ^{19}F).

To obtain spectra instead of images, frequency variations in the MR signal must be used to display the chemical shift information. Thus spatial encoding of the signal can no longer be performed by activating the frequency-encoding gradient as before. Different methods of spatial localization are therefore required for clinical spectroscopy than for routine MR imaging.

A second difference between MRI and MRS concerns the inherently poorer signal-to-noise ratio (SNR) of MRS. Because we are seeking to divide up the signal from each pixel into a number of smaller components (i.e., chemically distinct species), or because we are attempting to record nuclear magnetic resonance (NMR) spectra from nuclei such as ^{31}P (which are less abundant than ^1H), the SNR of spectra is poorer than that of MR images. To obtain an acceptable level of SNR in reasonable imaging times, much larger voxels are required for MRS than for routine imaging applications. In practice, spectroscopy studies typically use voxel sizes of 1 to 5 cm^3, whereas voxels for imaging are usually of size 1 to 5 mm^3.

Several spectroscopic localization methods are listed in Table 9-1. Unless one is involved in spectroscopy research, it is probably not too important to understand the many subtle variations among these. The reader should recognize, however, that despite recent advances, all these localization methods are imperfect. Spillover of spectra from one voxel into the next invariably occurs, and sometimes this spectral "contamination" may even arise from tissues far outside the volume of interest. Additionally, because of inhomogeneity-induced broadening of spectral linewidths, ambiguity in the identification of certain spectral lines may exist in some experiments. I thus caution you to evaluate clinical MRS papers cautiously when you encounter them in your readings; they remain full of traps and pitfalls in interpretation despite the best intentions of their authors.

Reference

Bottomly PA. The trouble with spectroscopy papers. JMRI 2:1, 1992.

Q 	How is hydrogen spectroscopy performed on a clinical MR imager?

In clinical MR imaging the signal from water protons overwhelms that emitted from the other chemical species. If the water peak is suppressed (e.g., by using CHESS or 1331 pulses, see Q 9.04), the signals from many interesting ^1H-containing molecules may be measured (Fig. 9-6). As discussed in Q 2.16 to Q 2.18, the chemical shift δ reference for hydrogen spectroscopy is tetramethylsilane (TMS), which is assigned a value $\delta = 0.0$.

Lactate ($\delta = 1.5$) is an important indicator of anaerobic metabolism and accumulates in tissues of patients with ischemia or hypoxia. Lactate measurements are thus important in the hydrogen spectroscopy of cerebrovascular accident (stroke). However, spillover of lipid resonances

TABLE 9-1. Localization Methods in Clinical Spectroscopy

Method	Description	Comments
STEAM (stimulated echo acquisition mode)	Application of three radiofrequency (RF) pulses that intersect as a cubic or rectangular volume; stimulated echo recorded	Excellent localization method with little outside "contamination," but only limited volumes can be recorded; useful for ^{1}H spectroscopy when combined with water suppression; relatively low signal-to-noise ratio; cannot be used with short T2 resonances (e.g., ^{31}P)
ISIS (image-selected in vivo spectroscopy)	Series of spatially selective 180° pulses that acquire free induction decay signals (FIDs) with and without inversion of spins; data subtraction performed	Widely used for ^{31}P spectroscopy because signals with short T2 times can be measured; versatile, can be combined with solvent suppression, inversion recovery, and spin echo techniques; drawbacks include specific absorption ratio limitations, motion sensitivity, necessity for accurate shimming, and spatial localization problems
CSI (chemical shift imaging)	FID phase encoded in each of desired dimensions without using readout gradient; Fourier transform (FT) produces frequency data used to construct spectra	Simultaneous acquisition of spectra from multiple regions; applicable to both ^{1}H and ^{31}DP; 1DFT, 2DFT, and 3DFT implementations possible; 3DFT limited by long imaging times and voluminous amounts of data
DRESS (depth-resolved surface coil spectroscopy)	Makes use of transmit-receive surface coil (having limited volume of excitation) with selective RF pulses and perpendicular magnetic field gradients	Useful for ^{31}P spectroscopy in superficial body regions amenable to surface coil examination (e.g., muscle); limited spatial selectivity; phase artifacts

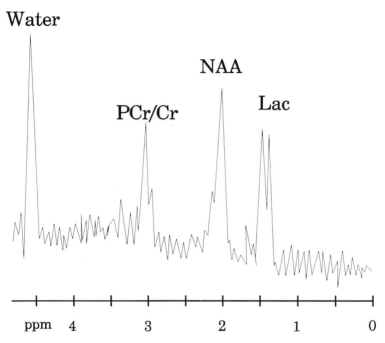

Fig. 9-6. ¹H spectrum from a region of ischemic brain showing a lactate *(Lac)* peak. *N*-acetylaspartate *(NAA)* and phosphocreatine/creatine *(PCr/Cr)* peaks are also seen. A small amount of water signal at 4.65 ppm has also leaked through despite its being supposedly saturated.

($\delta = 1.1$ to 1.6) may contaminate lactate spectra and make its validity questionable in superficial brain regions and in skeletal muscle.

N-acetylaspartate (NAA, $\delta = 2.0$) is found only in the brain and spinal cord. Its presence and level correlate crudely with neuronal integrity and the fraction of neuronal elements contained within neoplasms.

Phosphocreatine and creatine (PCr and Cr, $\delta = 3.0$) are involved in adenosine triphosphate (ATP) metabolism (see Q 9.09), and their combined hydrogen peak is useful as a reference level for other spectra. PCr is not found in the liver or kidney, and checking for a PCr peak in the spectra of these organs provides a method of quality control for evaluating the adequacy of spatial localization.

Other molecules that may be occasionally identified in water-suppressed ¹H spectroscopy include aromatic amino acids (tyrosine, histidine, tryptophan, $\delta = 6.0$ to 7.5), cholesterol (liver only, $\delta = 6.5$ to 8.0), brain/myelin–related amino acids (choline, taurine, glycine, $\delta = 3.0$ to 3.5), and liver-related amino acids (glutamate, aspartate, $\delta = 2.0$ to 3.0).

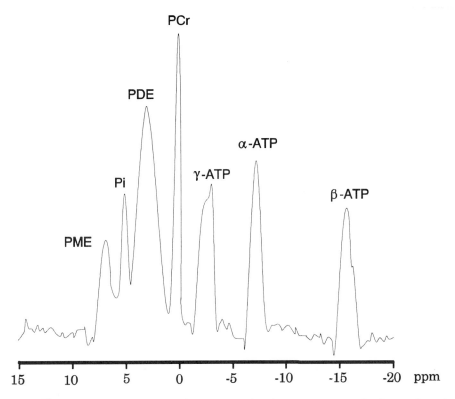

Fig. 9-7. ^{31}P spectrum from normal brain. Note the three separate peaks from adenosine triphosphate (ATP).

Q	How is phosphorus spectroscopy performed?
9.09	

After hydrogen, phosphorus is the next most important naturally occurring element of interest in biological MRS studies. The gyromagnetic ratio (γ) of ^{31}P is 17.2 MHz/T, resulting in a resonance frequency of 25.9 MHz at 1.5 T (compared with 63.9 MHz for ^{1}H). Furthermore, the natural abundance of ^{31}P is much lower than that of hydrogen, so that it generates a signal only about 1/20 as strong as that obtainable from ^{1}H. A typical ^{31}P spectrum from normal brain is shown in Fig. 9-7.

The reference value (chemical shift = 0) for in vivo ^{31}P NMR studies is generally taken to be PCr (phosphocreatine), which is stable under most conditions. In chemistry applications the P_i (inorganic phosphate) peak

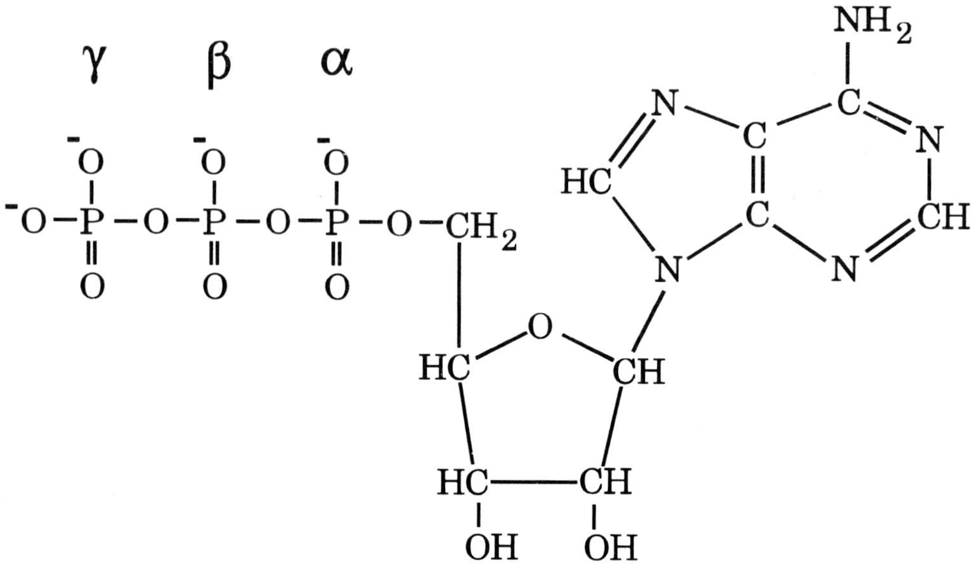

Fig. 9-8. The ATP molecule with labeling of the α, β, and γ phosphate moieties.

may be used instead as a reference (typically an 85% solution of ortho-phosphoric acid). The peaks in Fig. 9-7, labeled PME (phosphomonoesters) and PDE (phosphodiesters), are indicators of membrane synthesis and are usually elevated when a tumor is metabolically active. ATP (adenosine triphosphate) is the energy-containing compound essential for oxidative metabolism. The three separate peaks (α, β, and γ) represent signals from the three different phosphorus nuclei within this molecule (Fig. 9-8). PCr is a precursor in the formation of adenosine diphosphate (ADP) according to the following reactions:

$$PCr + ADP \rightarrow ATP + Cr$$

$$ATP \rightarrow ADP + P_i + Energy$$

Although the ADP concentration cannot be directly measured, it may be estimated from spectroscopic data by using the following relationship:

$$[ADP] \propto [P_i]/[PCr]$$

Tissue pH can be estimated by measuring the chemical shift between P_i and PCr. This relationship is nonlinear, but as an approximation, a 5 ppm chemical shift corresponds to about 0.5 pH unit.

Clinically, therefore, the greatest current use of ^{31}P spectroscopy seems to be in the evaluation of high-energy phosphate metabolism in metabolic disorders (McArdle's disease, muscular dystrophy, cardiomyopathy), ischemia (brain, heart, renal transplant), and tumor metabolism. Both prognosis and response to therapy may be predicted by ^{31}P spectroscopy in patients with some of these diseases.

Reference

Bottomley PA. Human in vivo NMR spectroscopy in diagnostic medicine: clinical tool or research probe? Radiology 170:1, 1989.

Q 9.10	**What is POMP?**

POMP (*p*hase-*o*ffset *m*ulti*p*lanar) imaging is a technique in which two separate slices are simultaneously excited by a composite RF pulse. This RF pulse is a multiplex of the individual RF pulses needed to stimulate each

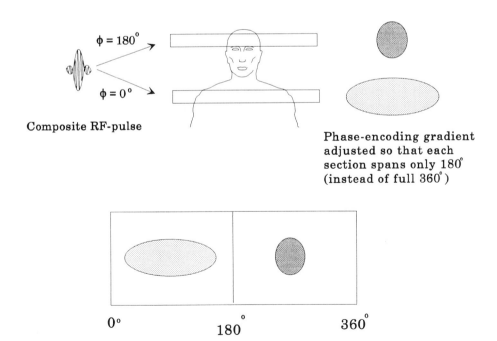

$\phi = 180°$

$\phi = 0°$

Composite RF-pulse

Phase-encoding gradient adjusted so that each section spans only 180° (instead of full 360°)

0°   180°   360°

Fig. 9-9. Phase-offset multiplanar (POMP) imaging. A complex RF pulse simultaneously stimulates two slices, which are phase offset from one another by an amount that depends on the phase-encoding step (here 180°).

of the two slices, phase shifted from each other so that the resulting images do not overlap (Fig. 9-9).

To distinguish between signal components from each of the two excited slices, the FOV in the phase-encoding direction must be doubled. This process is similar to that used in the no-phase-wrap technique (see Q 6.08). To preserve imaging time and SNR, the number of excitations is cut in half. The resultant data set then contains two images with the desired spatial resolution. The phase offset for the images and composite RF pulses will vary with the phase-encode step. At step 1, for example, the first image is phase encoded over a range of 0° to 180°, whereas the second image is encoded over a range of 180° to 360°.

Despite these theoretical advantages, POMP is hampered because certain forms of noise and phase-encoding artifacts (e.g., flow, wrap-around) may be propagated from one image to the other. Furthermore, because POMP cannot be used in conjunction with a no-phase-wrap option, it can only be applied in situations when the imaged object does not exceed the FOV in the phase-encode direction.

Reference

Glover GH. Phase-offset multiplanar (POMP) volume imaging: a new technique. JMRI 1:457, 1991.

| Q | **What is partial Fourier imaging?** |
| 9.11 | |

Partial Fourier imaging is a reconstruction method in which data from as few as one-half the normal number of phase-encoding steps are used to generate the entire MR image. This method reduces imaging time by up to 50% and is sometimes referred to as "½-NEX" or "fractional NEX" imaging. The term *½-NEX* is somewhat misleading, however, because what has been halved is the total number of phase-encoding steps (N_p), not the number of excitations per step (NEX). Other names for this technique include "phase conjugate symmetry" and "half Fourier imaging."

A full-resolution MR image can be reconstructed using only half the normal number of phase-encode steps because k-space is inherently symmetrical. This particular form of symmetry, known as *hermitian (conjugate) symmetry*, exists provided there are no phase errors across the

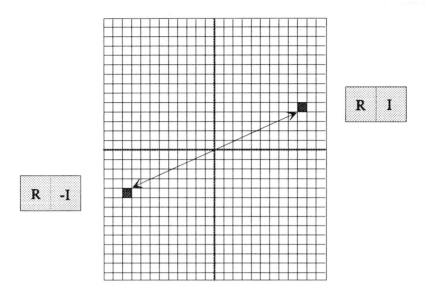

Fig. 9-10. Conjugate (hermitian) symmetry of k-space. Mirror image locations across the origin of k-space have real components of the same sign but imaginary components of the opposite sign.

sample. As shown in Fig. 9-10, the value of data points on one side of k-space can be calculated from values at mirror image locations across the origin. In other words, the signal intensity of a point on the rising portion of an echo obtained using a positive phase-encode step is the mirror image of that on the downward portion of another echo obtained using the corresponding negative phase-encode step.

All image data sets contain some phase errors, and therefore the conjugate symmetry approximations are not perfect. As commercially implemented, therefore, partial Fourier techniques require sampling of slightly more than half the lines of k-space (Fig. 9-11). These extra lines are then used to generate phase correction maps of k-space, allowing a more accurate prediction of missing values. Even better approximations can be obtained by sampling three fourths of k-space; this is sometimes called "¾-NEX imaging."

Although partial Fourier techniques reduce imaging time while preserving spatial resolution, this is accomplished at the expense of SNR. For ½-NEX imaging, SNR is reduced by a factor of $\sqrt{\frac{1}{2}}$, or about 70% compared with a conventional 1-NEX sequence.

References

Feinberg DA, Hale JD, Watts JC et al. Halving MR imaging time by conjugation: demonstration at 3.5 kG. Radiology 161:527, 1986.

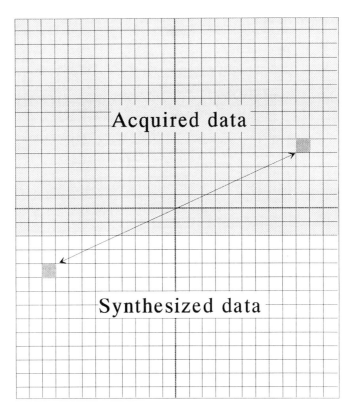

Fig. 9-11. Partial Fourier ("½-NEX") imaging samples a little more than half of k-space, restricting the number of phase-encoding steps. The other half of k-space is reconstructed by conjugate symmetry.

MacFall JR, Pelc NJ, Vavrek RM. Correction for spatially dependent phase shifts for partial Fourier imaging. Magn Reson Imaging 6:143, 1988.

Q 9.12	What is fractional echo imaging, and how does it differ from fractional NEX imaging?

Fractional echo imaging, also known as "read symmetry," is similar to the partial Fourier (½-NEX) techniques discussed in Q 9.11 in that only part of k-space is sampled and the remainder is calculated using properties of conjugate symmetry. In fractional echo imaging, however, all phase-encoding steps are acquired, but only part of each echo is sampled, generally the back half.

Why would one want to sample only part of an echo? The answer is that by sampling only part of an echo, the echo time (TE) can be made shorter

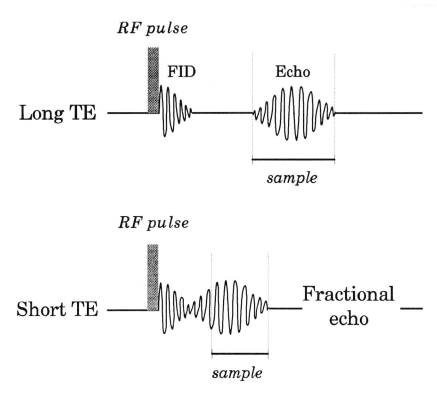

Fig. 9-12. When echo time (TE) is short, the free induction decay (FID) generated by the RF pulse may spill into the first part of the echo and interfere with its signal. Fractional echo techniques sample only the back half of each echo and reconstruct the front halves by read conjugate symmetry.

than would otherwise be possible. Being able to obtain extremely short TE values may be particularly advantageous in MRA, T1-SE, and fast GRE applications.

When TE is very short, part of the free induction decay (FID) signal generated by the preceding RF pulse may spill into the early rising portion of the echo (Fig. 9-12). By sampling only the back half of each echo and using read conjugate symmetry to extrapolate the front half, we obtain an image with short TE and little interference between the FID and echo signals. In terms of k-space, we are sampling the right half and calculating the left (Fig. 9-13).

| Q 9.13 | Why don't you combine the read conjugate symmetry and phase conjugate symmetry techniques? Then you could really save time by collecting only one-fourth the k-space data. |

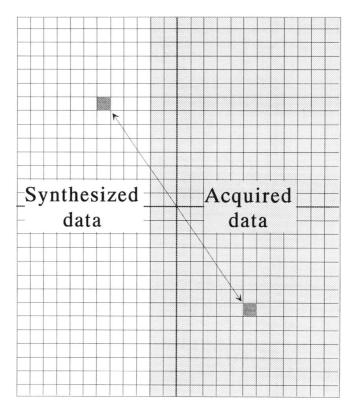

Fig. 9-13. K-space diagram of fractional echo imaging.

The symmetry of k-space relied on for success of the fractional echo and fractional NEX techniques is *diagonal* in nature. Collecting only one quadrant of k-space by combining the two techniques would allow one only to fill in the mirror image quadrant across the origin of k-space (Fig. 9-14). Therefore, the read conjugate and phase conjugate symmetry techniques cannot be used together; one fourth of k-space is not sufficient to reconstruct the entire image accurately.

| Q 9.14 | How does one obtain a rectangular field of view? |

A rectangular FOV can be obtained by sampling *alternate* phase-encode lines in k-space while leaving the maximum and minimum amplitudes of the phase-encoding gradient unchanged (Fig. 9-15). This process halves the

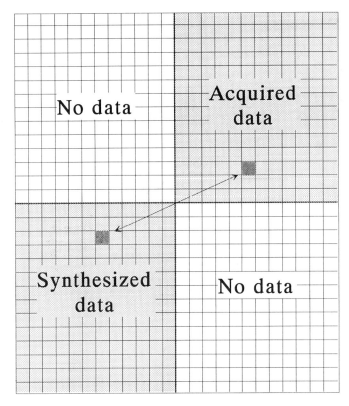

Fig. 9-14. K-space being "diagonally symmetrical" prevents one from imaging with only one quarter of the data.

number of phase-encoding steps (N_p), but doubles the *increment* between successive steps. From Q 4.06 we learned that

$$\text{Gradient area} \times (\text{FOV}_p / N_p) = \text{Constant}$$

Therefore, if the maximum gradient strength is unchanged and N_p is halved, the field of view in the phase-encode direction (FOV$_p$) must also be reduced by one-half. In other words, FOV$_p$ is inversely proportional to the increment between the phase-encoding steps. Doubling the increment, therefore, halves the FOV$_p$, resulting in a rectangularly shaped image. The FOV in the frequency-encode direction remains unaffected. Furthermore, because both the FOV$_p$ and N_p have been reduced by one-half, pixel size in the phase-encode direction (FOV$_p / N_p$) and overall spatial resolution of the image are also unchanged.

The rectangular FOV option is most beneficial in imaging the spine and

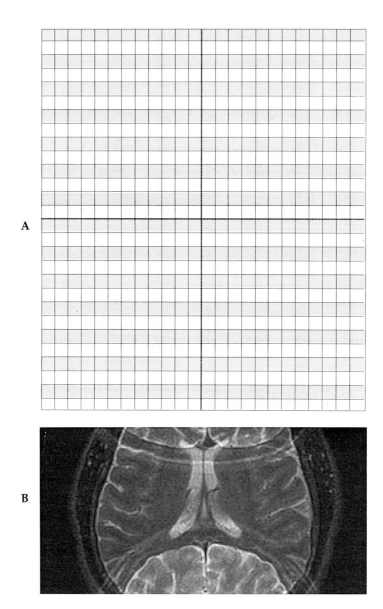

Fig. 9-15. **A,** Rectangular field of view (FOV) imaging samples alternate lines of k-space. **B,** Reconstructed brain image maintains spatial resolution, but FOV is cut in half. Note severe wraparound (aliasing) that has occurred because object was larger than ½ FOV.

extremities, where one anatomical dimension is much longer than the other. Some scanners allow adjusting the phase-sampling ratio over a large range; accordingly, considerable latitude may be permitted in the size and shape of the rectangular FOV.

Rectangular FOV techniques have two major problems, however. First, because fewer phase-encoding steps are acquired, SNR decreases. Second, because FOV_p has been reduced, wrap-around in the phase-encoding dimension may occur (Fig. 9-15, *B*). Careful positioning of the patient and the use of saturation bands may be needed to eliminate this wraparound artifact.

Q	**What is diffusion imaging?**

9.15

Molecular diffusion refers to the random, microscopic translational movement of water and other small molecules in a tissue caused by thermal processes (i.e., brownian motion). In a pure liquid the expected distance a molecule diffuses in time *t* can be modeled as a "random walk" with a gaussian distribution. Its variance is proportional to $6Dt$, where *D* is a proportionality constant known as the *diffusion coefficient*. Typical values for *D* in human tissue range from about 0.2×10^{-3} to 2.9×10^{-3} mm^2/sec.

In MR imaging the motion of water molecules by diffusion through a nonuniform magnetic gradient (*G*) results in an irreversible signal loss through intravoxel dephasing. This increased signal attenuation resulting from diffusion depends somewhat on the details of the pulse sequence used but in general has the form of an exponential decay [$\exp(-kD\,G^2\,TE^3)$] where *k* is a constant.

In routine MR imaging, diffusion effects contribute relatively little to overall signal intensity, causing signal attenuation of no more than 2%. However, it is possible to design sequences that are highly sensi-tive to diffusion effects. This is accomplished by applying strong pulsed gradients during evolution of the MR signal, which is gener-ated either by a long TE SE, GRE, or echo planar technique. Diffusion-sensitized images generally appear "T2 weighted" but with lower signal intensity from regions where diffusion is greatest. By using paired or interleaved sequences and varying the strength of the diffusion-sensitizing gradients, it is possible to measure apparent dif-fusion coefficients in tissues or to produce diffusion coeffi-cient maps of the tissue.

Diffusion-sensitive sequences have been shown to be clinically useful in the detection of early ischemic infarction when conventional T2-weighted images are negative. They have also been used to differentiate cysts from solid tumors, to measure deep body temperatures, and to study cerebrospinal fluid dynamics.

Limitations of diffusion-weighted imaging at present include restricted availability and specialized equipment requirements (e.g., high-strength gradients, echo planar capabilities.) Furthermore, diffusion images are frequently degraded by artifacts from eddy currents, flow, and gross patient motion.

Reference

Le Bihan D, Turner R, Moonen CTTW, Pekar J. Imaging of diffusion and microcirculation with gradient sensitization: design, strategy, and significance. JMRI 1:7, 1991.

Q 9.16	What is meant by a variable bandwidth technique?

Variable bandwidth (BW), also known as extending sampling, is a method now available on several major scanners to increase SNR in routine MR imaging. The basic concepts of SNR and receiver BW were considered in Q 4.13, where BW was defined to be the number of complex points sampled in an echo (usually 256 or 512) divided by the sampling time (typically between 8 and 64 msec). These parameters result in signal BWs of 4 to 32 kHz on most commercial scanners.

Extended sampling time is accomplished by reducing the amplitude of the readout gradient while prolonging its length (Fig. 9-16). This results in an echo that is "spread out" in time. In principle, since the SNR is proportional to the square root of the sampling time, doubling the sampling time (or halving the BW) should result in a 40% increase in SNR. This may be particularly advantageous on long TE images where the echo is weak.

As with all MR techniques promising increased SNR, the variable BW technique also has certain tradeoffs and disadvantages. First, longer sampling provides a longer window for unwanted spurious echoes to be detected. These may be manifest as rippling or zipperlike artifacts in the center of the image. The longer sampling window also gives more time for patient motion and flow artifacts to be generated. Secondly, chemical shift artifacts are accentuated using a narrow BW technique because a smaller band of frequencies spans each pixel. Similarly, magnetic field inhomogeneities and artifacts from ferromagnetic objects

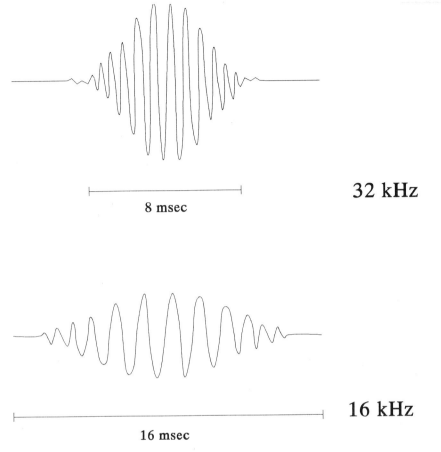

Fig. 9-16. Comparison of echoes recorded using bandwidths of 16 kHz and 32 kHz. The 16 kHz bandwidth echo is obtained by doubling the sampling time and halving the readout gradient amplitude.

are accentuated. This may result in greater geometric distortion and greater slice-to-slice differences in size.

Q 9.17 **What is fast spin echo imaging?**

Fast spin echo (FSE) imaging, also known as rapid SE or turbo-SE imaging, is a commercial implementation of the RARE (*r*apid *a*cquisition with *r*efocused *e*choes) technique, originally proposed by Hennig et al. This pulse sequence, illustrated schematically in Fig. 9-17, superficially resembles a routine multiecho SE sequence in that it uses multiple 180° refocusing

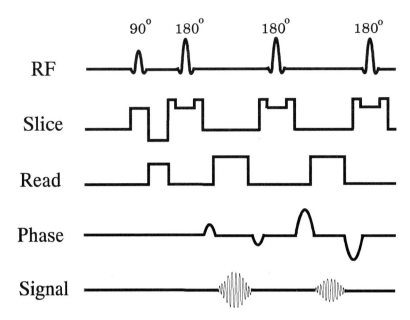

Fig. 9-17. The fast spin echo (FSE) pulse sequence. Each echo is obtained using a different phase-encoding step.

pulses after a single 90° pulse to generate a train of echoes. The FSE technique, however, changes the phase-encoding gradient for each of these echoes (the standard multiecho sequence collects all echoes in a train with the same phase encoding). As a result of changing the phase-encoding gradient between echoes, multiple lines of k-space (i.e., phase-encoding steps) can be acquired within a given repetition time (TR). The number of echoes acquired in a given TR interval is known as the *echo train length* (ETL), which typically ranges from 4 to 16. The *echo spacing* (ESP), or time between successive echoes, may also be adjusted, but is usually on the order of 20 msec.

Because multiple phase-encoding lines are acquired during each TR interval, FSE techniques may significantly reduce imaging time. When the number of slices is not the limiting factor, imaging time is inversely proportional to ETL. That is, an FSE sequence with an ETL of eight can be performed in one-eighth the time of a conventional SE sequence with the same TR.

Image contrast can be made to resemble that of a conventional SE technique by clustering the collection of low-order phase-encoding steps near the TE value desired. This may be done because global image contrast is determined principally from signals acquired at the low-order phase-encoding steps (the high-order steps contribute mostly to edge detail). Therefore, although each echo in a train has been acquired with a different

TE, the *effective TE* dictating overall image contrast is determined by the ET at which the low-order steps were performed.

Reference

Melki P, Mulkern RV, Panych LP, Jolesz FA. Comparing the FAISE method with conventional dual-echo sequences. JMRI 1:319, 1991.

Q 9.18	How do you select parameters, such as echo train length and echo spacing, in a fast spin echo sequence?

FSE techniques are undergoing constant refinement and variation, and therefore no one strategy can be considered optimal for all applications. Furthermore, clinical experience is still limited concerning which parameters may be best for imaging certain diseases. Despite these uncertainties, several general principles of FSE imaging are sufficiently well established to allow some useful guidelines to be determined in the selection of imaging parameters.

First, FSE techniques make possible the ability to obtain *within a reasonable time* images with very long TR and TE values (e.g., TR 4000, TE 120 msec). Such extremely long TR and TE values may be useful in certain applications (e.g., attaining a myelographic effect in spinal imaging, characterizing liver hemangiomas, visualizing inner ear structures). However, such extremely long TR/TE values may be *suboptimal* in many applications (e.g., routine brain imaging) when superior lesion detection is attained with medium-length TR and TE values (e.g., TR = 2000 to 3000, TE = 60 to 100).

Increasing ETL reduces acquisition time and increases signal homogeneity. However, it also results in a decrease in overall SNR and contrast-to-noise ratio (CNR) bacause the later echoes are weaker. The use of later echoes also produces more spatial blurring. This spatial blurring effect results from T2-related signal loss on late echoes; recall that these echoes are obtained with higher-order phase encodings corresponding to high spatial frequencies and details in the image.

Increasing ESP permits the use of longer TEs but adversely impacts SNR and contrast. Motion, susceptibility, and edge-related artifacts increase. In general, increased ESP has predominantly deleterious consequences on image quality; the shortest permitted ESP should therefore be chosen in most applications.

The number of slices required to cover an anatomical region in a given TR interval should also be considered in selection of ETL. In conventional two-dimensional Fourier tranform (2DFT) SE imaging, recall that the "dead time" at the end of each TR interval is not wasted; this time is used to excite other slices in the multislice acquisition (see Q 4.04). A tradeoff exists in FSE imaging between the ETL and the number of allowed slices for a given TR. If the ETL is too large, two separate FSE acquisitions (with double the imaging time) may be required to encompass the required number of sections.

Q 9.19	Why is fat excessively bright on fast spin echo images?

One of the most striking differences between conventional SE and fast SE imaging is the paradoxically higher signal from fat on FSE images. The physical basis of this phenomenon remains in dispute, although most investigators agree that *J*-coupling processes play an important role.

J-coupling, introduced briefly in Q 2.15, is a quantum-derived interaction between two nuclear spins on the same molecule resulting from "distortion" in their electron clouds. The strength of this interaction is described by the factor *J*, which for lipid protons has a value of 5 to 12 Hz. Unlike chemical shifts, which are proportional to the strength of the applied field, *J*-coupling interactions are independent of magnetic field strength. The small frequency shift caused by *J*-coupling produces a dephasing of nearby protons on lipid molecules during the evolution of the MR signal. For $J = 5$ to 12 Hz, maximum dephasing between *J*-coupled protons occurs at TEs of 25 to 100 msec. Therefore, when fat is imaged using a conventional SE sequence with TE of 25 to 100 msec, the additional dephasing caused by *J*-coupling shortens the measured T2 value and reduces signal intensity. A longer T2 value and relatively higher signal would be observed for TE greater than 100 msec or TE less than 25 msec. For ESPs less than 25 msec, the measured T2 of fat increases by up to 50% compared with conventional SE measurements using longer TE values.

In FSE imaging the closely spaced 180° pulses break up this pattern of *J*-modulation dephasing, although the *J*-coupling offset itself is not refocused by the 180° pulses. A complete understanding of this process requires a knowledge of quantum mechanics and is therefore well beyond the scope of this text. Nevertheless, this process can be understood in the sense that multiple 180° pulses, when applied at intervals shorter than $1/J$, render all *J*-coupled spins chemically "equivalent." The resultant signal is then no longer modulated by the coupling.

References

Henkelman RM, Hardy PA, Bishop JE et al. Why fat is bright in RARE and fast spin-echo imaging. JMRI 2:533, 1992.

Listerud J, Einstein S, Outwater E, Kressel HY. First principles of fast spin echo. Magn Reson Q 8:199, 1992.

 Q 9.20 **Are there any other differences in image contrast between conventional spin echo and fast spin echo imaging?**

In addition to the obvious brighter signal from fat seen in FSE imaging, several other subtle differences in contrast may be noted compared with conventional SE imaging.

First, because different phase-encoding steps are collected at different times, there may be subtle differences in contrast behavior between tissues with different T2 values. This phenomenon, known as *k-space filtering*, potentially may result in failure to detect small objects with T2 values close to background.

Subtle changes in the size of small objects may also occur in FSE imaging. This results from alteration of the image point-spread function in the FSE compared with conventional SE technique. This complex effect of k-space sampling may explain why certain edges appear excessively sharp and why nerve roots in the thecal sac are exceptionally well delineated on FSE images.

A third effect seen on FSE images is related to increased magnetization transfer and saturation effects. The multiple 180° pulses in FSE act as resonant-offset pulses, as in MT imaging (see Q 9.01). These MT effects cause a decrease in the signals of some stationary tissues, such as gray and white matter, compared with routine SE sequences. Conversely, cerebrospinal fluid and fat are not suppressed and appear somewhat brighter than brain matter.

Reference

Constable RT, Anderson AW, Zhong J, Gore JC. Factors influencing contrast in fast spin-echo imaging. Magn Reson Imaging 10:497, 1992.

Q	What is echo planar imaging?
9.21	

Echo planar imaging (EPI) is a method of ultrafast MR signal acquisition in which all k-space is sampled by rapid gradient reversals and echo collection after a single set of RF pulses (Fig. 9-18). Total planar imaging times as short as 30 to 40 msec are possible. EPI holds the promise of "real-time" MR imaging, and several companies are now testing EPI prototype systems at research sites.

The hardware requirements for an EPI system are severe. Gradient coils must be able to generate 20 to 40 mT/m fields with rise times less than 200 μsec. Analog-to-digital converters must have extremely rapid digitizing rates (high bandwidths), operating with sampling intervals of 1 to 4 μsec;

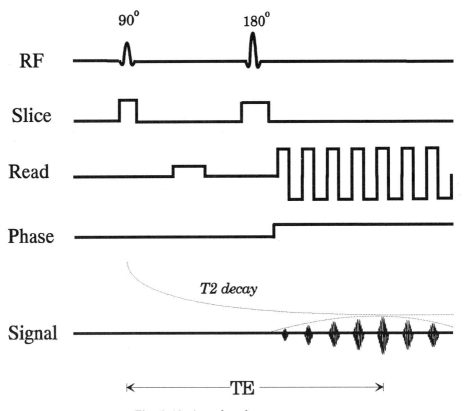

Fig. 9-18. An echo planar sequence.

appropriate computer memory must be available to store and process the voluminous amounts of data received. Chemical shift artifacts must be controlled by means of presaturation techniques. Acoustic noise must be mechanically damped. Flexible pulse programming tools must also be accessible to allow generation of various k-space trajectories: zigzag, rectangular, and spiral patterns.

Potential applications of EPI include functional (perfusion) imaging of the brain and heart, diffusion imaging, dynamic motion studies of the heart and gastrointestinal tract, and rapid time-resolved angiography. The extension of MR imaging to critically ill patients and nonsedated children also seems promising as EPI techniques are perfected.

Reference

Cohen MS, Weisskoff RM. Ultra-fast imaging. Magn Reson Imaging 9:1, 1991.

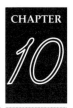
Safety and Biological Effects

Several years ago, I was shown a newspaper clipping from a super-market tabloid reporting an MR disaster in France. According to the story, a patient had a metal plate in his head as a result of previous injury and surgery. The MR technologists were unaware of this, however, and brought him into the scanner room. As soon as he was laid on the table, the magnetic field ripped out the plate from the top of his head, killing him instantly!

Such stories have become virtual "urban legends" in the MR world. In fact, just last month I heard a story about several people in France who were killed during the testing of an echo planar imaging system. Why these stories seem to originate in France I do not know, but they all reflect an anxiety about electromagnetism in general and misunderstandings about MR imaging technology in particular.

Nevertheless, there *are* some real dangers associated with magnetic fields, and anyone working with MR imaging devices should be aware of these. It *is* true that people with pacemakers have died during scanning, that metal objects have been propelled into scanners and injured people, and that thermal burns have occurred. So all this concern is not without foundation.

Here are your questions and my best answers about MR safety and biological effects. This last chapter is dedicated to those of you with *enquiring* minds.

Q **Many patients have metallic implants within their bodies that may cause problems during MR imaging. How do you screen for these?**

The detection and identification of metallic foreign materials within a patient before MR imaging is important because motion or displacement of these objects may result in injury. We rely principally on clinical history provided by the patients or their families to ascertain the presence of an implanted metallic foreign body. This is done in a purposely redundant fashion before the MR scan. In the waiting room, all patients are required to fill out a three-page medical history form that includes questions about prior surgeries, known implanted foreign bodies, occupation (e.g., sheet metal worker), and military service (possible bullets or shrapnel). In at least two places on the form, patients are specifically asked whether or not they have cerebral aneurysm clips, pacemakers, or metallic fragments within their bodies. Immediately before scanning, the technologist also asks the patient these same questions verbally.

Before entry into the scanning suite, patients must walk through an airport-style metal detector. This is not sufficiently sensitive to detect small objects within the body but is used to find external accoutrements such as hairpins and earrings that might be pulled loose when the patient is brought into the scanner.

Reference

Finn EJ, Di Chiro G, Brooks RA, Sato S. Ferromagnetic materials in patients: detection before MR imaging. Radiology 156:139, 1985.

Q **Which metallic implants are safe to scan, and which ones are not?**

Fortunately, the overwhelming majority of patients whose bodies contain biomedical implants, materials, and devices may safely undergo MR imaging. Although many implants contain metal and will create focal MR artifacts, only those with ferromagnetic properties (i.e., metals that are "magnetizable") will potentially move or rotate when placed in the scanner's magnetic field. Furthermore, only a small subset of these ferromagnetic devices will develop torques sufficiently great to create a medical hazard at fields less than 1.5 T.

In particular, nearly all orthopedic appliances (including joint prostheses, plates, screws, nails, and rods) are firmly imbedded within bone, and their presence is not a contraindication to MR imaging. Most neurosurgical devices (including shunts, drains, reservoirs, plates, and mesh) pose no hazard, and the vast majority of ocular, otologic, and dental implants are also safe. Hemostatic clips, wires, and drains used in all forms of surgery should generally cause no undue concern.

In general, it is easier to remember the relatively few devices *not* to scan. These include certain cerebral aneurysm clips, implanted electronic devices (e.g., pacemakers, cochlear implants), ferromagnetic shrapnel and bullets in critical locations (e.g., the eye), magnetically activated implants (tissue expanders, ocular prostheses), and several miscellaneous intravascular devices (e.g., Swan-Ganz catheters, recently placed inferior vena cava filters).

Reference

Shellock FG, Curtis JS. MR imaging of biomedical implants, materials, and devices: an updated review. Radiology 180:541, 1991.

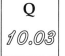

Q **What do you do if you find that a patient has a cerebral aneurysm clip?**

For many years the presence of a cerebral aneurysm clip was considered an absolute contraindication to MR imaging, for fear that the metallic clip might rotate or move within the field, shearing off the neck of the aneurysm with disastrous consequences. Today we recognize that many types of cerebral aneurysm clips are composed of nonferromagnetic metals and therefore will not move when placed within a magnetic field. Lists of MR-compatible and MR-incompatible aneurysm clips are available. Patients with nonferromagnetic cerebral aneurysm clips may be safely scanned, although one should expect to see an artifact several centimeters in diameter near the clip on MR images.

MR-compatible aneurysm clips have been used exclusively by neurosurgeons at our institution for the last 5 years, so generally we do not overly question the referral of one of their patients for MR imaging. For medicolegal and patient safety reasons, however, we do not scan patients with cerebral aneurysm clips referred from outside our institution unless at least one of the following conditions is met: (1) the patient is reliable and reports he or she has previously undergone MR scanning elsewhere without complications; (2) the referring physician sends a letter stating the exact name and model of the clip; or (3) I personally see a copy of the patient's medical record or operative note naming the type of clip.

Reference

Klucznik RP, Carrier DA, Pyka R, Haid RW. Placement of a ferromagnetic intracerebral aneurysm clip in a magnetic field with a fatal outcome. Radiology 187:855, 1993.

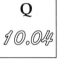

Q **What about other types of surgical clips, both intracranially and elsewhere?**

All surgical clips typically used for hemostasis (e.g., Hemoclips, Surgiclips) are nonferromagnetic, and patients with these clips may be safely scanned at any time regardless of clip location. Some skin staples are weakly ferromagnetic; they may create imaging artifacts but are nevertheless safe to scan. In patients with skin staples, I recommend covering the staples with a bandage so that they are not accidentally dislodged during imaging.

Reference

Shellock FG, Crues JV. High-field strength MR imaging and metallic biomedical implants: an ex vivo evaluation of deflection forces. AJR 151:389, 1988.

Q **Why is it that patients with cardiac pacemakers should never be scanned?**

Several theoretical and practical considerations necessitate the exclusion of any patient with a cardiac pacemaker from MR imaging. First, a pacemaker contains numerous magnetically and electrically sensitive electronic components that may potentially "short out" or be rendered nonoperational when placed in the scanner. Second, the magnetic field of the scanner may cause closure of the reed switch of the pacemaker, converting it from demand mode to asynchrony. Finally, electromagnetic currents induced by the scanner within the pacemaker leads could mimic the heart's normal electrical activity; this could potentially "fool" the sensing circuitry of a demand pacer and inhibit its proper output, even if the patient were asystolic. At least two deaths have been reported during the inadvertent MR imaging of patients with cardiac pacemakers.

Reference

Pavlicek W, Geisinger M, Castle L et al. The effects of nuclear magnetic resonance on patients with cardiac pacemakers. Radiology 147:149, 1983.

Q 10.06 | **Can you think of any other implanted electronic devices besides pacemakers that should not be placed in a magnet?**

Patients with automatic internal defibrillators, cochlear implants, implanted neural stimulators (including transcutaneous electrical stimulation [TENS] units and inductive thalamic stimulators), and bone-growth stimulators fall into this category. Patients with any of these devices should not undergo MR imaging. Out of similar theoretical concerns, we have traditionally not scanned patients with implanted infusion pumps at our institution; however, a recent report states that at least one brand of pump (SynchroMed) will not be damaged by clinical imaging at 1.5 T.

Reference

von Roemeling R, Lanning RM, Eames FA. MR imaging of patients with implanted drug infusion pumps. JMRI 1:77, 1991.

Q 10.07 | **What about patients with metal heart valves?**

Quite surprisingly, it is safe to scan nearly all patients with artificial heart valves, even metal ones. This is true even though some of these prostheses are mildly ferromagnetic and are deflected to variable degrees by the magnetic field. However, the magnetic torque experienced by these valves is small compared with the natural forces exerted on the valve by the beating heart itself.

A possible exception to this rule involves the pre–6000 series Starr-Edwards valves, which exhibit significantly stronger ferromagnetic deflection than other types. Starr-Edwards valves have a ball-in-cage design easily recognized on chest radiographs. Furthermore, because most were implanted before 1970, relatively few patients still have these in place. Soulen et al. have suggested that it is wise to refrain from imaging patients with such valves in magnets stronger than 0.35 T if there is any clinical question of valve dehiscence or integrity of the annulus.

Reference

Soulen RL, Budinger TF, Higgins CB. Magnetic resonance imaging of prosthetic heart valves. Radiology 154:705, 1985.

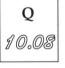

Q 10.08 I've heard that patients have been blinded by movement of intraocular metal fragments during MR imaging. How do you make sure that a patient doesn't have an orbital foreign body before imaging?

You are no doubt referring to a famous case from California in 1985 when a former sheet metal worker was blinded from motion of an occult intraocular metallic fragment during MR imaging. This metal fragment measured 2.0 × 3.5 mm and had been interpreted both on initial computed tomography (CT) and at ophthalmologic examination as a benign postinflammatory calcification, likely a previous parasitic *(Toxicara)* granuloma. On being removed from the scanner after successful MR imaging at 0.35 T, the patient experienced a tugging sensation in his eye, a flash of light, then a dramatic decrease in vision. Examination revealed massive vitreous hemorrhage and retinal laceration.

To screen patients for intraocular and intraorbital foreign bodies, we specifically ask them if they have any occupational or avocational exposure to metalworking and if they have ever been struck in the eyes or face by metal fragments. If the answer to either of these questions is "yes," we perform a plain film examination of the orbits before MR imaging.

Although some centers have advocated the use of orbital CT for this purpose, experimental evidence in cadavers has shown that the threshold size of metallic particle detection using CT (0.07 mm^3) is not remarkably superior to that of plain films (0.12 mm^3). Since it is unlikely that submillimeter particles from industrial sources will penetrate the sclera, plain film examination of the orbits in high-risk patients is cost-effective and probably is sufficient for the detection of metallic foreign bodies that pose a potential risk to the patient at MR imaging.

References

Kelly WM, Paglen PG, Pearson JA et al. Ferromagnetism of intraocular foreign body causes unilateral blindness after MR study. AJNR 7:243, 1986.

Otto PM, Otto RA, Virapongse C et al. Screening test for detection of metallic foreign objects in the orbit before magnetic resonance imaging. Invest Radiol 27:308, 1992.

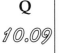

Q 10.09 | **Besides foreign bodies, are there any other eye-related potential hazards in MR imaging?**

Yes. Several immediately come to mind.

First, all eye makeup, especially mascara, should be removed before imaging. Such cosmetics often contain iron oxides that create a local artifact and may even result in eye irritation during MR imaging. Eyelid tattoos may create similar problems; one woman experienced painless local swelling of her eyes 4 hours after an MR examination.

Second, movement of eyelid palpebral springs may pose a potential risk to the patient, particularly if implanted as recently as 1 month before imaging. At least one model of retinal tack (Western European) is ferromagnetic, and patients with this implant probably should not undergo MR imaging.

Certain ocular prostheses are held in the orbit by magnets, and patients with these should not be placed in the scanner.

To my knowledge, patients with all types of intraocular lens implants may be safely scanned.

References

Albert DW, Olson KR, Parel JM et al. Magnetic resonance imaging and retinal tacks. Arch Ophthalmol 108:320, 1990.

Gangarosa RE, Minnis JE, Nobbe J et al. Operational safety issues in MRI. Magn Reson Imaging 5:287, 1987.

Seiff SR, Vestel KP, Truwit CL. Eyelid palpebral springs in patients undergoing magnetic resonance imaging: an area of possible concern. Arch Ophthalmol 109:319, 1991.

Q 10.10	**What about implants within the ear?**

As mentioned previously, cochlear implants may potentially be damaged by exposure to strong magnetic fields, and patients with these devices should not undergo MR imaging if the device is functional.

Virtually all middle ear prostheses are nonferromagnetic, with one exception (the McGee platinum–stainless steel piston produced during mid-1987). These prostheses have been recalled by the manufacturer (Richards Medical), and patients who received such implants have been issued warning cards not to undergo MR imaging. All ventilation tubes are made of either Teflon or titanium and will not be displaced in a magnetic field.

References

Applebaum EL, Valvassori GE. Further studies on the effects of magnetic resonance imaging fields on middle ear implants. Ann Otol Rhinol Laryngol 99:801, 1990.

Shellock FG, Schatz CJ. High-field strength MR imaging and metallic otologic implants. AJNR 12:279, 1991.

Q 10.11	**What about dental materials and devices?**

Many dental materials are ferromagnetic and create local artifacts during MR imaging but nevertheless pose no hazard to the patient. To minimize artifact, we have patients take out all removable bridgework before imaging. The only devices that should cause some concern are clad magnetic dental appliances; patients with these may be safely scanned after removal of the magnet-containing portion of the device.

Reference

Gegauf F, Laurell KA, Thavendrarajah A, Rosentiel SF. A potential MRI hazard: forces on dental magnet keepers. J Oral Rehabil 17:403, 1990.

Q 10.12	Can patients with an inferior vena cava (IVC) filter be safely scanned?

Yes, provided at least a month has elapsed since its placement, and there is no clinical suspicion of loosening or migration. In general, the same comments apply to other intravascular coils, filters, and stents. Although many such devices are ferromagnetic, the force of magnetic deflection at 1.5 T has been measured in vitro to be no greater than 8400 dynes (0.02 lb), which should not be sufficient to dislodge any of these devices, provided they are properly seated and incorporated into the vessel wall.

Reference

Teitelbaum GP, Bradley WG Jr, Klein BD. MR imaging artifacts, ferromagnetism, and magnetic torque of intravascular filters, stents, and coils. Radiology 166:657, 1988.

Q 10.13	I work in an inner-city hospital and see many patients with bullets, pellets, and other metallic shrapnel in their bodies. Is it safe to scan these patients?

The vast majority of bullets and pellets used in North America both for hunting and for Saturday night "entertainment" are composed of nonferromagnetic materials and are thus safe to scan. However, military shrapnel, as well as certain jacketed bullets used by police and drug dealers, is strongly ferromagnetic and therefore poses a theoretical risk to patients during MR imaging. Some BBs and shotgun pellets should also be included in this category.

The true risk posed by these ferromagnetic foreign bodies depends on their anatomical location, size, composition, orientation relative to the scanner field, and length of time since implantation. The movement of a ferromagnetic fragment is not a linear displacement but a rotation of the long axis of the foreign body to align with the magnetic field. Therefore, elongated objects oriented perpendicularly to the magnetic field lines are most likely to move. A round object (e.g., BB) does not experience any significant torque, even though it may be strongly ferromagnetic. The length of time since implantation is also an important factor in predicting potential injury; metallic fragments imbedded for years will likely be surrounded by fibrous scar tissue and thus be less likely to move.

The actual deflection forces of various ferromagnetic bullets have been measured in vitro, and the largest value (a military bullet from China) recorded was greater than 44.4×10^4 dynes. In English units, this is equivalent to a force greater than 1 pound. All other bullets tested had deflection forces of 2 ounces or less. Although a deflection force of 2 ounces experienced by a fragment imbedded subcutaneously or in skeletal muscle would likely be of trivial consequence, the same cannot be said if that fragment were imbedded in the orbit, spinal canal, or brain.

As a general approach to the problem of bullets, I first elicit a history from the patient concerning where, when, and with what type of gun the injury occurred. I then obtain a conventional radiograph of the area where the fragment is located to gain additional information concerning its size, shape, and precise location. In some cases, no bullet or radiopaque foreign body is found, despite the patient's insistence that a bullet is still there. More often only tiny metallic flecks are seen imbedded in bone or in the soft tissue; because of their small size, they should not contraindicate MR imaging, regardless of their composition.

If I ascertain that the bullet or shrapnel is likely to be ferromagnetic (as should always be presumed in veterans and those injured in times of war), I generally do not scan the patient if the object is imbedded in the brain, spinal canal, orbit, lung, mediastinum, or abdominal viscera. If the object is imbedded elsewhere and has been present for months to years, I generally proceed with scanning, provided the object is not large and elongated and is not near a vital neural or vascular structure. Even if I have decided that scanning poses minimum risk, I discuss with patients the remote possibility of injury and warn them to signal the technologist immediately if they experience any discomfort during the MR examination.

Reference

Teitelbaum GP, Yee CA, Van Horn DD et al. Metallic ballistic fragments: MR imaging safety and artifacts. Radiology 175:855, 1990.

Q 10.14	**Can you think of any other devices or clinical situations you haven't mentioned that might constitute a contraindication to MR imaging?**

Yes. I do not scan patients with Swan-Ganz thermodilution catheters because one patient has been reported in whom a portion of this catheter melted from eddy current heating.

Patients with certain external devices such as halo vests, Crutchfield tongs, and Hoffman fracture fixators should not be scanned, although MR-compatible versions of these devices now exist.

Although most carotid artery vascular clamps are safe, the Poppen-Blaylock variety is extremely ferromagnetic, and its presence is a contraindication to MR imaging.

Penile prostheses should generally elicit no concern, but one should realize that a single type (Dacomed Omniphase) is strongly ferromagnetic and may cause discomfort to a patient by its deflection at 1.5 T.

I prefer not to image patients with epicardial pacing wires still in place after cardiac surgery, not so much from a fear of inducing cardiac arrhythmias as from concern over the possibility of wire burns if this area is included in the region of radiofrequency stimulation.

Patients with certain magnetically activated tissue expanders have been deemed unsafe for MR imaging.

The reader should be aware than any metallic device, even one rigidly fixed to the skeleton and otherwise considered safe for MR imaging, may cause local tissue heating by an eddy current mechanism that may result in burns or discomfort. All patients with any type of implanted metallic device should therefore be made aware of such possible effects and told to notify the MR technologist immediately if any discomfort arises during the examination.

Reference

Shellock FG, Curtis JS. MR imaging of biomedical implants, materials, and devices: an updated review. Radiology 180:541, 1991.

| Q 10.15 | **How many of your patients are claustrophobic, and how do you handle them?** |

At our institution, approximately 2% of patients are unable to complete their MR examinations because of claustrophobia. Various interventions have been proposed to reduce the anxiety of such patients, none of which is entirely satisfactory. These maneuvers include providing patient education, blindfolding, piping in music, increasing air circulation and light within the scanner, allowing a family member to accompany the patient into the scanner, maintaining adequate verbal contact, providing mirrors or mirrored glasses, scanning patients in the prone position or inserting them feet first when possible, and applying various psychological desensitization techniques. We have tried and use all these methods from time to time, but we often rely on Valium for difficult patients.

Reference

Quirk ME, Letendre AJ, Ciottone RA, Lingley JF. Anxiety in patients undergoing MR imaging. Radiology 170:463, 1989.

Q 10.16	How do you sedate infants and children for MR imaging?

Proper sedation for infants and children in MR imaging is a compromise in that it involves obtaining a level of anesthesia that results in effective immobilization while minimizing the risks of significant respiratory depression and aspiration during the study. Heavy sedation during MR imaging carries a more significant risk than the equivalent level of sedation during CT or interventional procedures because the infant or child is located far within the bore of the scanner. Even with pulse oximetry and careful observation by a nurse, aspiration can occur during the procedure.

The first and most important aspect of sedating infants and children is to deprive them of sleep the night before. Parents or nurses should be instructed to keep the child up at least 2 hours beyond the usual bedtime at night and to awaken the child 1 to 2 hours earlier than usual in the morning. The MR examination ideally should be scheduled for midmorning or at the time of the child's usual nap. Clear liquids only are allowed within 4 hours of the anticipated sedation (except for infants, who may continue their usual feedings).

For infants and small children up to 25 kg, I prefer to use chloral hydrate by the oral or rectal route. In my opinion the most common reason for failure of this regimen is inadequate dosage. An initial dose of 75 mg/kg (up to a maximum of 2 g) should be administered, followed by an additional 25 mg/kg if the child is not asleep within 30 minutes.

For larger children, I occasionally first try a DPT cocktail (25 mg Demerol, 6.25 mg Thorazine, 6.25 mg Phenergan per ml) administered by deep intramuscular (IM) injection at a dose of about 1 ml/30 lb.

If chloral hydrate or DPT fails, further anesthesia with pentobarbital (Nembutal) may be attempted, although the physician should be cognizant of the added respiratory depressive effects when multiple drugs are used.

I prefer the intravenous route, since when sedation with this drug is indicated, it is wise to maintain a route for IV access. If the patient has not received other drugs, a loading dose of 5 mg/kg is administered, followed by supplementary doses of 2 mg/kg after 30 minutes, as needed. If this barbiturate regimen fails, we refer the patient for examination under general anesthesia.

Reference

Boyer RS. Sedation in pediatric neuroimaging: the science and the art. AJNR 13:777, 1992.

Q 10.17	How do you monitor anesthetized or critically ill patients during an MR scan?

A wide variety of MR-compatible monitoring devices are now available (Table 10-1). For lightly sedated patients, we generally use only a pulse oximeter; for those more heavily sedated or prone to apneic episodes, we use both a pulse oximeter and a capnocytometer. Patients undergoing general anesthesia are monitored with a pulse oximeter, capnocytometer, blood pressure cuff, and precordial stethoscope.

TABLE 10-1. MR-Compatible Monitoring Devices

Device Type	Company	City
Pulse oximeter	In Vivo Laboratories, Inc.	Broken Arrow, OK
	Nonin Medical, Inc.	Plymouth, MN
Capnocytometer	Biochem International	Waukesha, WI
	Puritan-Bennett Corp.	Los Angeles, CA
Respirator	Ohio Medical	Madison, WI
	Columbia Medical Marketing	Topeka, KS
	Monaghan Medical Corp.	Plattsburgh, PA
Blood pressure monitor	In Vivo Laboratories, Inc.	Broken Arrow, OK
Temperature monitor	Luxtron	Mountain View, CA
Skin perfusion monitor	Vasomed, Inc.	St. Paul, MN
	Medpacific Corp.	Seattle, WA
Stethoscope	Anesthesia Medical Supplies	Santa Fe Springs, CA

MR-compatible anesthesia machines and respirators are also available. Alternatively, the usual MR-incompatible versions of these devices may still be used if placed outside the scanner room and connected to the patient by long hoses. For low-field installations, these devices may even be located in the scanner room several feet from the scanner, as long as they are secured to the floor or wall.

An important point is that electronic monitoring devices are no substitute for the physical presence of a nurse or technologist in the scanner room while an anesthetized or sedated patient is undergoing MR imaging. Some crises, such as aspiration of gastric contents, may occur repeatedly over several minutes before the oxygen saturation levels drop enough to set off the pulse oximeter alarm. Such potential medical disasters may be easily averted if the patient is kept under the watchful eye of a skilled health care provider during the MR examination.

Q 10.18	Are there any special considerations one must be aware of when setting up a patient for a cardiac-gated MR study?

Yes. Several considerations relate to the proper handling of cables and wires associated with the electrocardiographic or photoplethysmographic apparatus. Electrical currents that may be induced in these cables can cause subsequent heating and patient burns if proper procedures are not followed. In particular, the technologist should:

- Never cross cables and wires. Avoid bending cables more than 180° and forming loops.
- Remove leads from the patient and cables from the table during ungated scans.
- Route wires and cables down the center of the magnet bore, under the cushion and away from the patient.
- Always place foam insulation between the patient and a wire or cable.

Q 10.19	How loud is the MR scanner? Should patients wear earplugs?

The pulses of electrical current that flow through the gradient coils and adjacent conductors during MR scanning result in significant vibrations and a loud banging sound. The amplitude of this noise is in the range of

65 to 95 dB, depending on the pulse sequence selected. The most noise is generated by rapid gradient echo sequences. In one series, 43% of patients without ear protection experienced transient mild loss of hearing after routine MR imaging. Permanent hearing loss has occasionally been reported.

All patients should therefore be given earplugs or headphones during routine MR imaging to prevent transient or permanent hearing loss.

Reference

Brummett RE, Talbot JM, Charuhas P: Potential hearing loss resulting from MR imaging. Radiology 169:539, 1988.

Q **Does MRI pose any risk to the developing fetus? Do you scan pregnant patients?**

No consistent or convincing body of evidence has yet been assembled to suggest that short-term exposure to electromagnetic fields (e.g., the exposure that occurs during MR imaging) harms the developing fetus. The reader should be aware, however, that in a few studies, *prolonged* exposure to electromagnetic radiation has been linked with some deleterious effects on embryogenesis, chromosomal structure, or fetal development. Such positive studies purport to have demonstrated accelerated cleavage in sea urchin embryos, lower birth weights in rats, chromosomal aberrations in human lymphocyte cultures, altered bacterial mutation rates, modulation of mitosis frequency in slime molds, and malformations of chick and frog embryos. Nevertheless, many more studies have failed to demonstrate any measurable harmful effects of electromagnetic fields on animal or human embryos. Therefore, at present, no *conclusive* scientific evidence supports a direct relationship between MR exposure and disorders of embryogenesis. Of course, no one has proved that small or subtle effects do not occur.

For this reason, we do not cavalierly recommend MR imaging in pregnant patients, particularly if there is no overpowering clinical necessity for the scan or if an equivalent nonionizing diagnostic technique (e.g., ultrasound) will suffice. Despite these cautions, we do not hesitate to scan a pregnant patient when we believe such a study is medically indicated. Reasonable indications for an MR scan during pregnancy might include a herniated disk, pituitary dysfunction, or suspected brain tumor.

For medicolegal purposes, either I or one of my resident physicians talks personally with the patient and obtains informed consent for imaging. We explain the concepts expressed in the first paragraph: that there are no *proven* harmful effects of MR imaging on the fetus but that the risk may not be zero. We also inform each patient that any alternative radiological diagnostic tests (e.g., CT, myelography) would likely require using x-rays, and we believe the risks of exposing the developing fetus to x-rays is no less, and is probably greater, than the theoretical risks of MR imaging.

The use of gadolinium in pregnant and lactating women is discussed in Q 8.15.

Reference

Beers GJ. Biological effects of weak electromagnetic fields from 0 Hz to 200 MHz: a survey of the literature with special emphasis on possible magnetic resonance effects. Magn Reson Imaging 7:309, 1989. (A fascinating review concerning possible biological effects of electromagnetic fields, even including theories about ESP and military experiments with microwaves on humans in the former Soviet Union.)

Q 10.21	**What do you do about pregnant technologists?**

Although there is no definitive evidence that occupational exposure to MR-level magnetic fields may be harmful to a pregnant technologist or her fetus, I do recommend reduced exposure throughout pregnancy. It has been our policy to keep pregnant technologists out of the scanner rooms, at least during the first trimester. This practice minimizes their exposure to the higher level of static magnetic fields and eliminates completely their exposure to the time-varying (RF) fields. If a technologist has strong feelings about her occupational exposure during pregnancy, we assign her a clerical position far away from the scanner (a job we refer to as "tech-retary"). Fortunately, other jobs in the MR suite, such as patient preparation and counseling, image archiving, and filming, involve little or no magnetic field exposure.

Reference

Kanal E, Gillen J, Evans JA et al. Survey of reproductive health among female MR workers. Radiology 189:395, 1993.

Q 10.22	I've heard that the MR scanner changes one's EKG. Is this dangerous?

When a patient is placed in the magnetic field of an MR scanner, an elevation of the T wave of the electrocardiogram (EKG) is frequently noted. This elevation may be so marked that the T wave actually becomes larger than the QRS complex and causes faulty triggering in a cardiac-gated study.

This magnetic field effect on the EKG does not originate in the heart itself but represents a superimposed voltage within blood in the proximal aorta that has been induced by its flow in the magnetic field. The induction of a voltage in a conductive fluid flowing through a magnetic field is a well-known effect in magnetohydrodynamics. This is the same principle by which electromagnetic blood flowmeters operate. In humans imaged at 1.5 T, this induced voltage is on the order of 10 mV. This voltage is superimposed on the T wave because this is the time of maximum flow in the proximal aorta. This induced low voltage distorts the EKG but produces no untoward effects on the heart or blood flow. It is therefore only a curious phenomenon and not an effect of clinical significance.

Reference

Tenforde TS, Budinger TF. Biological effects and physical safety aspects of NMR imaging and in vivo spectroscopy. In Thomas SR, Dixon RL, eds. NMR in medicine: instrumentation and clinical applications. Medical monograph no 14. New York: American Association of Physicists in Medicine, 1985, p 493.

Q 10.23	What is SAR?

SAR stands for *specific absorption rate* and is a measure of the amount of energy deposited by a radiofrequency (RF) field in a certain mass of tissue. The units for SAR are therefore given in watts per kilogram (W/kg).

For a homogeneous sphere of tissue of radius r and conductivity σ placed in an MR scanner of field strength B_o, both the average and the peak SAR are proportional to the square of the RF flip angle (α). Specifically:

$$SAR \propto \sigma\, r^2 B_o^2\, \alpha^2\, D$$

The variable D represents the *duty cycle*, which is the percentage of time in an imaging sequence in which the RF pulses are applied.

The reader should note several features about SAR that follow directly from this equation. First, because SAR is proportional to the square of field strength, it is significantly greater in high-field scanners. Second, since SAR is proportional to the square of the RF flip angle, 180° pulses deposit four times as much energy as do 90° pulses. Third, if the duty cycle is high (i.e., many RF pulses in a short time), the SAR will be greater. Finally, in the human body, electrical conductivities (σ) vary by a factor of 10, being smallest for tissues with low water content (e.g., fat, bone marrow) and highest for tissues with high water content (e.g., brain, blood, liver, cerebrospinal fluid). Focal "hot spots" with SAR deposition up to 2.5 times greater than predicted by this equation may occur if the imaged tissue is nonspherical or inhomogeneous (as the human body always is).

Current Food and Drug Administration (FDA) guidelines require MR imagers to generate SARs that do not exceed 0.4 W/kg (whole-body average) or 8.0 W/kg (within any single gram of tissue). For head imaging, an average SAR of up to 3.2 W/kg is acceptable. The 0.4 W/kg limit for whole-body indications was derived from animal studies in which the threshold for behavioral change (i.e., work stoppage) was found to be 4.0 W/kg. The 0.4 limit was chosen by the FDA as a factor of 10 lower than this threshold value for animals.

All MR imagers sold in the United States are required to have autosensing circuitry to limit the average SAR to meet FDA guidelines. Certain choices of imaging parameters may therefore not be allowed in scanner software if they would result in RF energy deposition that would exceed FDA limits. SAR limits often may be exceeded when saturation pulses or high duty cycles (short echo time, multiple slice) are used. Fast spin echo sequences, with their multiple 180° pulses, generate particularly high SAR values. Gradient echo sequences, using low–flip angle pulses and gradient reversals for signal refocusing, typically generate small SAR values.

Reference

Schaefer DJ. Safety aspects of magnetic resonance imaging. In Wehrli FW, Shaw D, Kneeland BJ, eds. Biomedical magnetic resonance imaging: principles, methodology, and applications. New York: VCH, 1988, p 553.

Q 10.24

Are any unique biological effects noted in the 4.0 T experimental scanners?

In human subjects undergoing MR imaging at 4.0 T, several biological effects are noticeable that are generally not present at 1.5 T. First, some patients experience dizziness and nausea after prolonged exposure or rapid head movement within the field. This effect is thought to result from motion of otoliths in the inner ear, which contain ferrite (ironlike) materials. A second effect is the generation of magnetophosphenes, small flashes of light caused by retinal discharges with rapid eye motion. The nerves of the palate are also stimulated by moving the head in such a field. Both magnetophosphenes and palatal nerve stimulation are probably caused by the motion-induced generation of eddy currents in the conducting tissue.

Although these effects are of little concern for patient safety, in my opinion they are reminders that we may be pushing the limits of acceptable magnetic field exposure for diagnostic imaging purposes.

References

Barfuss H, Fischer H, Hentschel D et al. Whole-body MR imaging and spectroscopy with a 4-T system. Radiology 169:811, 1988.

Schenck JF, Dumoulin CL, Redington RW et al. Human exposure to 4.0-Tesla magnetic fields in a whole-body scanner. Med Phys 19:1089, 1992.

Q 10.25

Are any unique biological effects seen in echo planar imaging?

Echo planar imaging systems introduce another variable into the realm of biological effects: those attributable to rapidly changing gradient fields. These effects are sometimes called "dB/dt effects," after the calculus notation representing the time rate of change of **B**. According to Faraday's law of induction, a changing magnetic field will generate a voltage and current in a conductor (e.g., the human body) directly proportional to dB/dt.

In conventional MR imaging, dB/dt values are in the range of 1 to 5 T/sec, and no biological effects directly related to this phenomenon have been observed. When dB/dt is increased to about 60 T/sec, however, human volunteers have noted muscular twitches in the face and back and uncomfortable "electric shock" sensations in the same areas. Because of these data, the FDA currently recommends that dB/dt not exceed 20 T/sec, which is a factor of three below those levels producing peripheral nerve stimulation. Theoretical calculations predict that the dB/dt thresholds for seizures and cardiac arrhythmias are an order of magnitude greater than that required for peripheral nerve stimulation.

Reference

Cohen M, Weisskoff R, Rzedzian RR, Cantor HL. Sensory stimulation by time-varying magnetic fields. Magn Reson Med 14:409, 1990.

Q	**Is it safe to live under power lines or sleep under an electric blanket at night?**

A growing body of scientific evidence suggests that prolonged exposure to 50 to 60 Hz magnetic fields may increase the risk of cancer. Several studies have demonstrated that children who live near power lines and adults whose occupations expose them to high electromagnetic fields (e.g., linemen, electrical workers) have an increased risk of leukemia, brain tumors, and other neoplasms. Even electric blankets and household appliances such as electric shavers and washing machines have come under scrutiny as possible environmental hazards.

Although many of these reported studies contain methodological flaws and a causative link between long-term electromagnetic exposure and cancer has not been fully established, these data should not receive a cursory dismissal. How, then, should we live and act in light of this present scientific uncertainty? For personal and policy decisions regarding the risks of exposure to electromagnetic fields, the concept of "prudent avoidance" put forth by Morgan and colleagues may be useful. Under this doctrine, one should incorporate the present level of evidence concerning the probable risks of electromagnetic exposure into decision-making processes, such as one's choice of home or job. Based on present studies, for example, at worst case, living under power lines may increase the risk of childhood cancer from 1 in 10,000 to 3 in 10,000 per year. This degree of increased risk should be incorporated into an array of factors used to make decisions concerning what constitutes an acceptable health risk in daily living. Other decisions (e.g., those concerning smoking, exercise, or diet) may prove much more important in determining one's overall health risk than whether one chooses to work in a magnet factory or sleep under an electric blanket at night.

As for me, I live far away from overhead power lines but still fearlessly maintain my office in the MR center at about the 3 gauss line. I shave each morning with an electric razor and do not think twice about standing near the microwave oven to watch my bowl of soup heat up for lunch. And on cold winter nights, I sleep next to my wife, Jeanine, under a soft, nonelectric blanket and a comforter. Not for philosophical or scientific reasons—I just like it that way.

References

Adey WR. Tissue interactions with nonionizing electromagnetic fields. Physiol Rev 61:435, 1981.

Florig HK, Hoburg JF. Power frequency magnetic fields from electric blankets. Health Phys 58:493, 1990.

Savitz DA. Power lines and cancer risk. JAMA 265:1458, 1991.

Appendix

The MR imaging literature is replete with abbreviations, acronyms, Greek letters, and other obscure symbols. This list translates some of the more common ones you may encounter. (ACR Glossary refers to the American College of Radiology. Glossary of MR terms, ed 3. Reston, Va: ACR, 1991.)

α	Alpha	Symbol used for RF flip angle
β	Beta	Symbol used for RF precession (resonant offset) angle
γ	Gamma	Symbol used for gyromagnetic ratio
δ	Delta	Symbol used for chemical shift
κ	Kappa	Symbol for magnetic susceptibility (SI)
μ	Mu	Symbol used for magnetic dipole; also used for magnetic permeability
ρ	Rho	Symbol used to denote spin density
σ	Sigma	Symbol used for conductivity
τ	Tau	Symbol often used to denote time delay between RF pulses
ϕ	Phi	Symbol used for phase
χ	Chi	Symbol used for susceptibility
ψ	Psi	Symbol used for wave function
ω	Omega	Symbol used for angular frequency
ω_o	Omega$_o$	Symbol used to denote the resonance (Larmor) frequency
AC	Alternating Current	Generic term, defined in ACR Glossary

ADC	Analog-to-Digital Converter	Generic term, defined in ACR Glossary
AFP	Adiabatic Fast Passage	Generic term, defined in ACR Glossary
B, B_o, B_1	—	Designation for magnetic field vectors (boldface) or their magnitudes (italics)
BW	Bandwidth	Generic term for range of frequencies transmitted or recieved (See Q 4.13)
CE	Contrast en-hanced	Generic term, defined in ACR Glossary
CE-FAST	Contrast-Enhanced FAST	Steady-state GRE technique with refocusing of the FID part of the signal (See Q 5.16); same as PSIF
CE-FFE-T1	Contrast-Enhanced Fast Field Echo with T1 weighting	Acronym for gradient-spoiled GRE sequence used by Philips; same as Siemens FLASH
CE-FFE-T2	Contrast-Enhanced Fast Field Echo with T2 weighting	Acronym for CE-FAST technique used by Philips
CGS	Centimeter-Gram-Second	System of measurement (See introduction to Chapter 1)
CHESS	Chemical Shift Selection	
CISS	Constructive In-terference in the Steady State	Acronym used by Siemens for technique combin-ing flow compensation with DESS signal
CNR	Contrast-to-Noise Ratio	Generic term, defined in ACR Glossary
COPE	Centrally Or-dered Phase Encoding	A respiratory compensation technique (See Q 6.12)
CORE	COnstrained RE-construction	Method of reconstructing artifact-free superreso-lution images
CPMG	Carr-Purcell-Meiboom-Gill	Method used in SE imaging in which phase of RF is varied between pulses (See Q 2.22)
CSFSE	Contiguous-Slice Fast-acquisition Spin Echo	FSE/RARE variant
CSI	Chemical Shift Imaging	Generic term, defined in ACR Glossary
CW	Continuous wave	Early NMR technique
dB	Decibel	Generic term, defined in ACR Glossary
dB/dt	Time derivative of B	Rate of change of magnetic field with respect to time
DC	Direct Current	Generic term, defined in ACR Glossary

DE	Driven Equilibrium	Generic MR technique using RF pulses to return flipped magnetization back to longitudinal direction; used in conjunction with MP-GRE sequences for T2 weighting (See Q 5.18)
DEFAISE	Dual-Echo Fast-Acquisition Interleaved Spin Echo	Double-echo variant of RARE
DESS	Double-Echo Steady State	Acronym used by Siemens for technique combining FISP and PSIF signals
DTPA	Diethylenetriamine pentaacetic acid	Chelating agent of gadolinium used in Magnevist (See Q 8.11)
E-SHORT	SHORT with SE/STE sampling	Elscint term for PSIF/CE-FAST technique
EPI	Echo Planar Imaging	Generic term, defined in ACR Glossary (See Q 9.21)
EPR	Electron Paramagnetic Resonance	MR phenomenon involving electrons; same as ESR
ESP	Echo SPacing	Time between echoes in a FSE sequence (See Q 9.17)
ESR	Electron Spin Resonance	MR phenomenon involving electrons; same as EPR
ETL	Echo Train Length	Number of echoes per TR in FSE sequence (See Q 9.17)
f	Frequency	Generic term (See Q 1.15)
F-SHORT	SHORT with FID sampling	Elscint term for FISP/GRASS sequence
FADE	FASE Acquisition Double Echo	True FISP technique sampling both FID and SE/STE components of steady-state signal
FAME	Fast-Acquisition MultiEcho	Acronym for FSE/RARE technique used by Picker
FASE	FAst Spin Echo	FSE/RARE variant
FAST	Fourier-Acquired steady STate	Acronym used by Picker for a steady-state GRE sequence similar to GRASS and FISP
FATE	Fast-TE	Same as FADE
FE	Field Echo	Alternative name for a gradient echo; generic term, synonymous with GE
FEDIF	Field Echo—DIFference	Acronym used by Picker for GRE sequence with water and fat signals out of phase
FEER	Field Even Echo by Reversal	Steady-state GRE sequence acronym used by Picker
FESUM	Field Echo—SUMmation	Acronym used by Picker for GRE sequence with water and fat signals in phase
FFE	Fast Field Echo	Steady-state GRE sequence acronym used by Philips

FFT	Fast Fourier Transform	Efficient computational method for performing a Fourier transform
FGR	Fast GRASS	Rapid GRE sequence acronym used by GE Medical
FID	Free Induction Decay	Generic term for MR signal occurring after an RF pulse (See Q 2.19)
FISP	Fast Imaging with Steady-state Precession	Steady-state GRE sequence acronym used by Siemens (See Q 5.14)
FLAIR	FLuid Attenuated Inversion Recovery	IR technique using long TI value to null signal from liquids
FLARE	Fast Low-Angle Recalled Echoes	FSE/RARE variant using low flip angles
FLASH	Fast Low-Angle SHot	Original name for steady-state incoherent GRE sequence developed by Haase and Frahm; commercial name used by Siemens for their gradient-spoiled GRE sequence (See Q 5.08)
FOV	Field Of View	Generic term, defined in ACR Glossary
FRE	Field Reversal Echo	Same as GRE
FSE	Fast Spin Echo	Acronym for RARE technique used by GE Medical (See Q 9.17)
FSPGR	Fast SPoiled GRASS	Similar to Turbo-FLASH
FT	Fourier Transform	Generic term, defined in ACR Glossary (See Q 4.01)
G	Gradient strength	Generic term, defined in ACR Glossary (See Q 1.05)
G	Gauss	Unit of magnetic field strength (See Q 1.01)
Gd	Gadolinium	Elemental symbol (See Chapter 8)
GE	Gradient Echo	Generic term (See Q 5.01)
GFE	Gradient Field Echo	Hitachi term for any GRE sequence
GMN	Gradient Moment Nulling	Flow compensation technique (See Q 7.10)
GRASE	GRadient And Spin Echo	Hybrid fast imaging technique using multiple GREs and SEs
GRASS	Gradient-Recalled Acquisition in the Steady State	
GRE	GRadient Echo	Generic term (See Q 5.01)
GRECHO	Gradient-Recalled ECHO	Resonex term for GRE
HFI	Half Fourier Imaging	Sampling only part of k-space and using phase conjugate symmetry to fill in the rest (See Q 9.11)

HYBRID	—	Fast imaging technique using both static and oscillating PE gradients, thus combining features of both FSE and EPI
Hz	Hertz	1 cycle per second
I	—	Nuclear spin quantum number (See Q 2.02)
IR	Inversion Recovery	Generic term, defined in ACR Glossary
J	—	Coupling constant (See Q 2.15 and Q 9.19)
kHz	Kilohertz	1000 hertz
LASE	Low-Angle Spin Echo	Large flip angle SE technique similar to THRIFT (see Q 5.05)
M	Magnetization	Designation for magnetization vector (boldface) or its magnitude (italics)
MAST	Motion Artifact Suppression Technique	Acronym for gradient moment nulling used by Picker
MHz	Megahertz	10^6 cycles per second
MIP	Maximum Intensity Projection	Method of generating MRA image from raw data
MOTSA	Multiple Overlapping Thin-Slab Acquisition	MRA technique (see Q 7.14)
MP-GRE	Magnetization-Prepared rapid GRE	Generic term proposed by Elster for any rapid GRE sequence using preparatory pulses
MP-RAGE	Magnetization-Prepared RApid Gradient Echo	3DFT implementation of Turbo-FLASH using preparatory pulses (See Q 5.18)
MPGR	Multiplanar GRASS	Acronym for general-purpose GRE sequence used by GE Medical
MR	Magnetic Resonance	Generic term, defined in ACR Glossary
MRA	Magnetic Resonance Angiography	Generic term, defined in ACR Glossary
MRI	Magnetic Resonance Imaging	Generic term, defined in ACR Glossary
MRS	Magnetic Resonance Spectroscopy	Generic term, defined in ACR Glossary
MT	Magnetization Transfer	Generic term (See Q 9.01)
MTR	Magnetization Transfer Ratio	Measure of signal change resulting from an MT pulse (See Q 9.01)
NEX	Number of EXcitations	Term used by GE Medical to denote the number of signals averaged for each phase-encoding step

NMR	Nuclear Magnetic Resonance	Generic term, defined in ACR Glossary
NPW	No Phase Wrap	GE Medical abbreviation for phase oversampling technique (See Q 6.08)
NSA	Number of Signals Averaged	Generic term to denote the number of signals averaged for each phase-encoding step
PC	Phase Contrast	Signal variations in flow caused by phase changes; an MRA method exploiting this phenomenon (See Q 7.06 and Q 7.12)
PE	Phase Encode	Generic term, defined in ACR Glossary
POMP	Phase-Offset MultiPlanar	RF multiplexing technique used by GE Medical to acquire multiple slices simultaneously (See Q 9.10)
ppm	Parts per million	Generic term, defined in ACR Glossary
PS	Partial Saturation	Generic term, defined in ACR Glossary
PSIF	"Mirrored" FISP	Acronym for steady-state GRE sequence with sampling of the SP/STE component used by Siemens
Q	—	Symbol used for bulk flow (See Q 7.01)
QUEST	QUick Echo Split imaging Technique	FSE variant using multiple unequally spaced RF pulses and collecting STEs and SEs
R-SE	Rapid Spin Echo	Generic term proposed by Elster for any RARE/FSE technique
RACE	Real-time ACquisition and velocity Evaluation	1DFT method of velocity measurement (See Q 7.15)
RAM-FAST	Reduced Acquisition Matrix FAST	Turbo-FLASH-like sequence used by Picker
RARE	Rapid Acquisition with Refocused Echoes	Original fast spin echo technique described by Hennig, acquiring multiple RF echoes with different phase-encoding steps (See Q 9.17)
Re	Reynold's number	Parameter used to estimate turbulence (see Q 7.03)
RF	RadioFrequency	Generic term, defined in ACR Glossary
RF-FAST	RadioFrequency-spoiled FAST	Acronym for RF-spoiled GRE sequence used by Picker
RICE	Rapid Imaging using Composite Echo	Acronym for FSE/RARE technique used by Toshiba
ROAST	Resonant Offset Averaged Steady State	Generic term proposed by Haacke for any steady-state coherent GRE sequence such as FISP/GRASS
ROPE	Respiratory Ordered Phase Encoding	Respiratory compensation technique (See Q 6.12)

SAR	Specific Absorption Rate	Measure of absorbed energy from MRI (See Q 10.23)
SE	Spin Echo	Generic term (See Q 5.01)
SI	Système International d'Unites	System of measurement (See introduction to Chapter 1 and Q 1.01)
SNR	Signal-to-Noise Ratio	Generic term (See Q 4.13)
SP-GRE	Spoiled GRE	Generic term proposed by Elster for any spoiled GRE sequence
SPGR	SPoiled GRASS	Acronym for RF-spoiled GRE sequence used by GE Medical
SS-GRE-FID	Steady-State GRE with FID sampling	Generic term proposed by Elster for sequences such as FISP/GRASS
SS-GRE-SE	Steady-State GRE with SE/STE sampling	Generic term proposed by Elster for PSIF/CE-FAST sequences
SSC	Steady-State Coherent	Generic term proposed by Haacke for any steady-state GRE sequence in which both nonzero longitudinal and transverse components develop
SSFP	Steady-State Free Precession	Name for any GRE sequence in which a nonzero steady state develops for both transverse and longitudinal components of magnetization; acronym used by GE Medical to refer to this sequence when the SE/STE is sampled
SSI	Steady-State Incoherent	Generic term proposed by Haack for spoiled GRE sequences
STAGE	Small Tip Angle Gradient Echo	Acronym used by Shimadzu for their general-purpose GRE technique
STE	STimulated Echo	Generic term (See Q 2.24)
STEAM	STimulated Echo Acquisition Mode	Imaging/spectroscopy technique using stimulated echoes (See Q 9.07 and Table 9-1)
STEP	STimulated Echo Progressive imaging	T1-weighted variant of RARE
STERF	STEady-state Refocused Free induction decay	Acronym used by Shimadzu for their sequence resembling PSIF
STIR	Short TI Inversion Recovery	Generic term (See Q 9.05)
T	Tesla	Unit of magnetic field strength
T1	—	Longitudinal relaxation time (See Q 2.09)
T2	—	Transverse relaxation time (See Q 2.10)
T2*	T2-star	Effective T2 relaxation time (See Q 2.12)
TE	Echo Time	Generic term, defined in ACR Glossary

THRIFT	Throughput Heightened Rapid Increase Flip T2	Picker acronym for large flip angle SE technique (See Q 5.05)
TI	Inversion Time	Generic term, defined in ACR Glossary
TMS	Tetramethylsilane	Reference compound for hydrogen spectroscopy (See Q 2.17)
TOF	Time-Of-Flight	Signal variations caused by inflow or outflow; an MRA method exploiting this phenomenon (see Q 7.05 and Q 7.12)
TR	Repetition Time	Generic term, defined in ACR Glossary
TSE	Turbo Spin Echo	Acronym for FSE/RARE technique used by Siemens/Philips
Turbo-FLASH	Turbo version of FLASH	Rapid GRE variant of FLASH used by Siemens
Turbo-SHORT	Turbo version of SHORT	Acronym for Turbo-FLASH-like sequence used by Elscint
VENC	Velocity ENCoding	Parameter that must be specified for phase contrast MRA (See Q 7.13)
VINNIE	Velocity imaging in cine mode	2DFT method of velocity measurement (See Q 7.16)

Index

A

Active shielding, 69
Active shimming, 67
Adenosine diphosphate (ADP), phosphorous
  spectroscopy and, 222
Adenosine triphosphate (ATP)
  hydrogen spectroscopy and, 220
  phosphorous spectroscopy and, 221-222
Aliasing, 145-151
  frequency, 152-154
  velocity, VENC and, 184
Aliasing artifacts, frequency-encode direction
  and, 152-154
Aliphatic lipid protons, T1 and T2 values and,
  42-43
Aliphatic protons, chemical shifts of, 50
Allergic respiratory disorders, 194
Amplitude of sine wave, 19-22
Anesthesia machines, MR-compatible, 253
Anesthetized patients, monitoring of, during
  MR scan, 252-253
Aneurysm clips, 242-243
Angiography
  black blood, 188
  magnetic resonance; see Magnetic resonance
    angiography
Angular frequency, 19-22
Anisotropy, chemical shift, T1 and T2 and, 48
Antialiasing, technique of, 151-152, 153
Antialiasing software, 151
Aorta, ascending, blood flow velocities in, 163
Aromatic amino acids, hydrogen spectroscopy
  and, 220
Aromatic proteins, chemical shifts of, 50-51
Arteriovenous fistulas, blood flow velocities in,
  163
Artifacts
  aliasing, 152-154
  central point, 159, 160-161
  chemical shift; see Chemical shift artifact(s)
  crisscross, 160, 161
  ghost; see Ghost artifacts
  Gibbs, 142-144
  herringbone, 160, 161
  motion; see Motion artifacts
  MR, 134-161
  phase, 172-173
  phase wraparound, 145-151
  ringing, 142-144
  spectral leakage, 142-144
  susceptibility, 145, 146, 147
  truncation, 142-144
  wraparound, 152-154
  zipperlike, 159-160

Ascending aorta, blood flow velocities in, 163
Aspiration of gastric contents during MR scan,
  253
Aspirin allergy, Gd-DTPA/dimeglumine and, 194
Asthma, Gd-DTPA/dimeglumine and, 194
Automatic internal defibrillators, 244
Avoidance, prudent, electromagnetic fields and,
  258-259

B

Bandwidth (BW)
  receiver, 89, 107-108
  RF transmitter, 89, 107
Bar magnet, magnetic dipole and, 15
Barbiturates for infants and children, 251-252
"Basic Principles of Magnetic Resonance Imag-
  ing," 79
BBs, MR imaging and, 248-249
Biological effects of MR imaging, 240-260
Black blood angiography, 188
Bladder, pseudolayering of gadolinium in, 192, 193
Blankets, electric, safety of, 258-259
Bloch equation, 33-36, 53
Blood, flowing
  accentuation of signals from, by GRE pulse
    sequences, 171-172
  spatial misregistration of refocused signal
    from, 178-181
Blood flow, 162-163, 165-166
  determination of direction of, 178-181
  slow, distinguishing thrombus from, 172-174
Blood pressure cuff for patient, 252-253
Blood velocities, usual, 163
Blood vessels, MR signal observed in, 166, 167
Boltzmann constant, 29
Bone-growth stimulators, MR imaging and, 244
Bowel MR contrast agents, 205-206
Brain, MR parameter weighting indices for, at
  0.35 T, 111
Brain-related amino acids, hydrogen spectros-
  copy and, 220
Breast milk, excretion of Gd-DTPA in, 205
Bridgework, dental, MR imaging and, 247
Brightness of vessel in MR imaging, 165-166
Brownian motion, 231
Bulk flow, measurement of blood flow in vessel
  and, 162-163
Bullets, MR imaging and, 242, 248-249

C

Capnocytometer, 252-253
Carbon, chemical shift of, 50
Cardiac gating in reduction of ghost artifacts,
  157-158

Cardiac pacemakers, 242, 243-244
Cardiac-gated MR study, 253
Carotid artery vascular clamps, 250
Carr-Purcell-Meiboom-Gill (CPMG), 58
Catheters, Swan-Ganz thermodilution, 249-250
Center frequency, setting, during prescan, 76-77
Centimeter-gram-second (CGS) system, 1
Central point artifacts, 159, 160-161
Centrally ordered phase encoding (COPE) in reduction of ghost artifacts, 157-158
Cerebral aneurysm clips, 242-243
Cerebrospinal fluid (CSF), accentuation of signals from, by GRE pulse sequences, 171-172
Chemical exchange, T1 and T2 and, 47
Chemical shift anisotropy, T1 and T2 and, 48
Chemical shift artifact(s), 134-141
Chemical shift imaging (CSI), 219
Chemical Shift Selection (CHESS), fat suppression and, 210, 212, 213, 218
Chemical shifts, 49
  free induction decay and, 53
  measurement of, 49-50
  prediction of, based on molecule's chemical structure, 50-52
  between water and fat protons, 138-139
Children
  gadolinium for, 197, 198
  sedation of, 251-252
Chloral hydrate for infants and children, 251
Cholesterol, hydrogen spectroscopy and, 220
Chopper method, fat suppression and, 210, 212
Chromosomal structure, effect of prolonged exposure to electromagnetic radiation on, 254-255
Clad magnetic dental appliances, 247
Claustrophobia, interventions for, 250-251
Cochlear implants, MR imaging and, 242, 244, 247
Coherent steady-state sequences versus incoherent steady-state sequences, 126-127
Coil tuning, 76
Compass needle
  frequency of oscillation of, 16, 17, 18-19
  magnetic dipole and, 15
  motion of, within magnetic field, 16, 17
Compression devices in reduction of ghost artifacts, 157-158
Conjugate symmetry, 224-225, 226
Contrast agents
  iodine, 196, 203
  magnetic resonance; *see* Magnetic resonance (MR) contrast agents
Contrast-enhanced FAST (CE-FAST), 132
Contrast-to-noise ratio (CNR) in fast spin echo imaging, 235
Corsets in reduction of ghost artifacts, 157-158
Cosmetics, eye, MR imaging and, 246
CPMG; *see* Carr-Purcell-Meiboom-Gill
Creatine (Cr), hydrogen spectroscopy and, 220
Crisscross artifacts, 160, 161
Critically ill patients, monitoring of, 252-253

Cross-relaxation, T1 and T2 and, 47-48
Cross-talk, 84-87
Crutchfield tongs, MR imaging and, 250
Cryogens, 64-65
Crystal double group, 32
Cyclic frequency, 19, 20

D

Dacomed Omniphase penile prosthesis, 250
Data clipping, 77, 78
dB/dt effects, echo planar imaging and, 258-259
Defibrillators, automatic internal, 244
Demerol, Thorazine, and Phenergan (DPT) cocktail in sedation of infants and children, 251
Dental materials and devices, 242, 247
Dephase lobe, 88
Dephase-rephase technique, 187
Dephasing, odd echo, 166, 174, 175
Depth-resolved surface coil spectroscopy (DRESS), 219
Deshielded protons, 49
Diamagnetism, 7-8, 10, 11-12
Diethylenetriamine pentaacetic acid (DTPA)
  gadolinium and, 189
  Magnevist and, 200
Diffusion coefficient, 231
Diffusion imaging, 48, 231-232
Dipole, magnetic, 15-16
  dipole-dipole interactions and, 44, 45-46
Dipole-dipole interactions, 16, 37, 44-48
Distal aorta, blood flow velocities in, 163
Dixon method, fat suppression and, 210, 211-212
Dotarem; *see* Gd-DOTA
DPT cocktail; *see* Demerol, Thorazine, and Phenergan cocktail
Drains, MR imaging and, 242
Driven-equilibrium (DE), 133
DTPA-BMA (bismethylamide), gadodiamide and, 201
Duty cycle, specific absorption rate and, 256
Dysprosium (Dy), paramagnetism of, 12

E

Ear implants, MR imaging and, 242, 244, 247
Earplugs, worn during MR imaging, 254
Echo planar imaging (EPI), 238-239
  biological effects and, 258-259
  chemical shift artifacts and, 139
Echo spacing (ESP) in fast spin echo imaging, 234, 235-236
Echo time (TE), fractional echo imaging and, 226-227
Echo train length (ETL) in fast spin echo imaging, 234, 235-236
Eddy currents, 68-69
Electric blankets, safety of, 258-259
Electric shavers, safety of, 258-259
Electricity and magnetism, basic principles of, 1-21
Electrocardiogram (EKG), effect of MR scanner on, 255-256

Electromagnetic blood flowmeters, magnetohydrodynamics and, 256
Electromagnetic fields, prudent avoidance and, 258-259
Electromagnetic radiation, prolonged exposure to, effect of, on fetus, 254-255
Electromagnetism, fundamental units of, 9
Electronic monitoring devices, 252-253
Embryogenesis, effect of prolonged exposure to electromagnetic radiation on, 254-255
Energy levels, Zeeman, quantum mechanics and, 24-25, 26-28
Enhancement, 166, 167, 168
Entry phenomenon, fresh blood flowing into volume of tissue and, 166
Epicardial pacing wires, MR imaging and, 250
Ernst angle, 115-116, 120
Even echo rephasing, 166, 174-176
Exchange coupling, ferromagnetism and, 13
Excitation, slice-selective, 82-84
Exorcist in reduction of ghost artifacts, 157-158
Extended matrix software, phase wraparound artifacts and, 151
Extending sampling time, 232, 233
Eye makeup, MR imaging and, 246
Eyelid palpebral springs, MR imaging and, 246
Eyelid tattoos, MR imaging and, 246
Eye-related hazards in MR imaging, 245-246

F

Faraday's law of induction, 258-259
Fast spin echo (FSE) imaging, 233-237
Fat, brightness of, on fast spin echo images, 236-237
Fat saturation pulses, 77, 140
Fat suppression, 210-217
  elimination of chemical shift artifacts in routine spin warp imaging and, 140
"Fat-sat" pulse; *see* Frequency-selective RF pulse
Feedthrough, zipperlike artifacts and, 159-160
Ferric ammonium citrate (Geritol) as GI contrast agent, 205-206
Ferrites as liver MR contrast agents, 206-207
Ferromagnetic bullets, 248-249
Ferromagnetic properties of metallic implants, 241
Ferromagnetism, 10, 11
  versus paramagnetism and superparamagnetism, 12-14
Fetus, risk to, of MR imaging, 254-255
Field echo, 117
Field of view (FOV)
  frequency-encoding gradient and, 88-89
  rectangular, 101, 228-231
  wraparound and, 145-151
Field-focused nuclear magnetic resonance (FONAR), 97
FISP versus PSIF, 131-132
Fistulas, arteriovenous, blood flow velocities in, 163

FLASH, 119, 126
  versus Turbo-FLASH, 132-133
FLASH bands, 123, 124
Flip angle, 114-115
  RF, 30
Flip angle pulse, low, 128
Flip-flop, 39, 40
Flow compensation (flow comp), 176-178
Flow eddies, vortex flow and, 165
Flow phenomena and MR angiography, 162-188
Flow void, turbulently flowing fluids and, 166
Flowmeter, electromagnetic blood, magnetohydrodynamics and, 256
Flow-related enhancement, fresh blood flowing into volume of tissue and, 166, 167
Fluorescence, spontaneous emission of energy and, 29
Flux density, 9
Foreign bodies, orbital, movement of, during MR scan, 245-246
Fourier imaging, partial, 224-225, 226
Fourier transform (FT), 79-82
Fourier-acquired steady-state (FAST), 68
Fractional echo imaging, versus fractional NEX imaging, 226-227, 228
Fractional NEX imaging, 224-225
Free induction decay (FID), 52-53, 61
  fractional echo imaging and, 227
  versus spin echo, 53-56
  steady-state free precession and, 122-125
Free induction (FID) sampling, steady-state GRE with, 118
Frequency, 19-22
Frequency aliasing, 152-154
Frequency encoding, 87-89, 97, 178-181
Frequency wraparound, 152-154
Frequency-encode direction, motion artifacts and, 155
Frequency-encoding gradient, 88, 89
Frequency-encoding gradient strength, 89
Frequency-selective fat suppression techniques, 210, 212-214
Frequency-selective RF ("fat sat") pulse, fat suppression and, 210, 212-214
Friction, oscillation of compass needle and, 18

G

Gadodiamide (Omniscan), 194, 200, 201, 202, 203
Gadolinium (Gd) based contrast agents, 200-202
  concentration of, pseudolayering and, 192, 193
  effect of, on T1 and T2, 190-191
  given to pregnant or lactating women, 205
  ionic, 200-202, 203
  MR contrast agents based on, 189-202
  nonionic, 200-202, 203
    renal tolerance of, 199
  paramagnetism of, 12
  renal failure or insufficiency and, 199-200
  T1- and T2-shortening effects of, 191-193
  use of, in pregnant and lactating women, 255
Gadopentetate dimeglumine, 200, 201

Gadoterate meglumine (Gd-DOTA), renal failure and, 199-200
Gadoteridol (ProHance), 200, 201, 202, 203
  high-dose regimens of, 204-205
  safety of, 194, 203
Gaseous helium, escape of, during quench, 66
Gaseous nitrogen, escape of, during quench, 66
Gastrointestinal MR contrast agents, 205-206
Gating, cardiac or respiratory, in reduction of ghost artifacts, 157-158
Gauss (G), 2
Gaussian system, 1
Gd-DOTA (Dotarem), 201, 202
Gd-DTPA/dimeglumine (Magnevist), 200, 201, 202, 206
  as bowel MR contrast agent, 206
  dosage of, 198-199
  hemodialysis and, 200
  for infants and children, 197, 198
  mean elimination half-life of, 196
  pharmacokinetics of, 196-197
  for pregnant or lactating women, 205
  relaxivities of, 191
  safety of, 194, 203
  severe reactions to, 195-196
Geritol; *see* Ferric ammonium citrate
Ghost artifacts, 155-158, 172-173
Gibbs artifacts, 142-144
Gradient coils, 5
Gradient echo (GRE), 61, 117
  magnetization-prepared, 118, 132-133
  versus spin echo, 112-113
  spoiled; *see* Spoiled GRE
  steady-state, with free induction decay sampling, 118
Gradient echo (GRE) imaging, 112-133
  chemical shift artifacts and, 140-141
  fat suppression and, 212
Gradient echo (GRE) pulse sequences, classification and nomenclature of, 117-118
Gradient moment nulling (GMN), 176-178
Gradient motion rephasing (GMR), 176-178
Gradient shielding, 69
Gradient spoiling, 119
Gradient-recalled echo, 117
Gradients
  MR scanners and, specifications for, 67
  shielded, eddy currents and, 68
GRASS/FISP sequences, 171, 127-130
Gyromagnetic ratio, 16, 24, 33

H

Haacke, Mark, 126
Hahn echo, 55, 56, 59
Half Fourier imaging, 224-225
1/2-NEX imaging, 224-225, 226
Halo vests, MR imaging and, 250
Hardware, MR scanner, 62-78
Harmonics, decomposition of triangular waveform by Fourier methods into, 79-80, 81
Hearing loss, earplugs or headphones worn during MR imaging to prevent, 254

Heart valves, metal, MR imaging and, 244-245
Helium
  gaseous, escape of, during quench, 66
  liquid, in superconducting MR scanners, 65
Hemoclips, 243
Hemodialysis, gadolinium-based contrast agents and, 199-200
Hemostatic clips, MR imaging and, 242, 243
Hepatic MR contrast agents, 206-207
Hermitian symmetry, 224-225
Herringbone artifacts, 160, 161
Heteronuclear coupling, 48
High-field MR scanners, 62-63
High-velocity signal loss, 167-168, 169
Hitachi MRP-5000, 64
Hoffman fracture fixators, MR imaging and, 250
Homospoil technique of fat suppression, 212
Horizontal-field magnets, 3, 4
  saddle coils and, 63
Hydrogen protons in water molecule, nuclear paramagnetism of, 12
Hydrogen spectroscopy, 218-220

I

Ice, T1 value of, 37
Iliac vessels, blood flow velocities in, 163
Image noise, white, 107, 108
Image selected in vivo spectroscopy (ISIS), 219
Imaginary MR signal channels, 71-72, 73-74
Imaging
  chemical shift, 219
  diffusion, 48, 231-232
  echo planar; *see* Echo planar imaging
  fast spin echo; *see* Fast spin echo imaging
  fractional echo, 226-227, 228
  fractional NEX, 224-225, 226-227
  gradient echo; *see* Gradient echo imaging
  1/2-NEX, 224-225, 226
  magnetization transfer, 208-210, 237
  partial Fourier, 224-225, 226
  phase-offset multiplanar, 223-224
  rapid spin echo, 233-235
  spin echo; *see* Spin echo imaging
  spin warp, 139-140
  3/4-NEX, 225
  turbo-SE, 233-235
Impedance matching, coil tuning and, 76
Implanted electronic devices, 242, 244
Implanted neural stimulators, 244
Implanted transfusion pumps, 244
In phase MR signal channels, 71-72
In quadrature MR signal channels, 71-72
Incoherent steady-state sequences versus coherent steady-state sequences, 126-127
Incremental phase contribution, 174-176, 177
Induced emission of energy, 29-30
Inductive thalamic stimulators, 244
Infants
  MR contrast agents for, 197, 198-199
  sedation of, 251
Inferior vena cava (IVC) filters, 242, 248
Inflow enhancement, 167, 168

In-plane pixel size, 101, 104
Intermediate field MR scanners, 62
Intermolecular dipole-dipole interaction, 37
Internal defibrillators, automatic, 244
Intramolecular dipole-dipole interaction, 37
Intraocular lens implants, MR imaging and, 246
Intraocular metal fragments, movement of, during MR scan, 245-246
Intraorbital foreign bodies, movement of, during MR scan, 245-246
Iodine contrast agents, 196, 203
Ionic Gd-based contrast agents, 200-202, 203
Ionic iodine contrast agents, 203
Iron, magnetic memory of, 13
Iron oxides in eye makeup, 246
Isochromat, spin, 25-26, 55
Isovue-300, osmolar load from, 203

J

J-coupling interactions, T1 and T2 and, 47
J-coupling processes, brightness of fat on fast spin echo images and, 236-237

K

Keller, Paul, 79
K-space, 98-101, 102-103, 104, 105-106
    in echo planar imaging, 238-239
    fractional echo imaging and, 226-227, 228
    partial Fourier imaging and, 224-225
    read conjugate symmetry and, 227-228, 229
    rectangular field of view and, 228, 229, 230
K-space filtering in fast spin echo imaging, 237

L

Lactate, hydrogen spectroscopy and, 218, 220
Lactating women, gadolinium-based contrast agents given to, 205
Ladder coils, 75
Laminar flow, 163-165
Lanthanide series of elements, gadolinium and, 189
Larmor frequency, 16, 25, 27, 28, 30-32, 35, 37, 39, 41, 58
Lattice, T1 relaxation and, 37
Lens implants, intraocular, 246
Linearly polarized transmit/receive coils for MR imaging, 70-71
Liquid helium and liquid nitrogen in superconducting MR scanners, 65
Liver MR contrast agents, 206-207
Liver-related amino acids, hydrogen spectroscopy and, 220
Localization methods in clinical spectroscopy, 218, 219
Longitudinal relaxation time, 37
Loudness of MR scanner, 253-254
Low-field MR scanners, 62-64

M

Magic angle, dipole-dipole interactions and, 45, 48
Magnet field homogeneities, 66-67
Magnet susceptibility, 9-11
Magnetic dipole, 15-16
    dipole-dipole interactions and, 44, 45-46
Magnetic dipole moment, 15
Magnetic domains, ferromagnetism and, 13
Magnetic field, 1-3, 6-9
Magnetic field gradient, 5, 6
Magnetic field intensity, 6, 9
Magnetic field strengths used for MR imaging, 62-63
Magnetic flux density, 6
Magnetic fringe field specifications, 67
Magnetic induction, 6
Magnetic induction field, 6, 9
Magnetic memory, ferromagnetism and, 13
Magnetic properties of matter, 10, 11
Magnetic resonance angiography (MRA), 23
    eddy currents and, 68
    flow phenomena and, 162-188
    magnetization transfer imaging and, 209
    time of flight, magnetization transfer imaging and, 209
Magnetic resonance (MR) artifacts, 134-161
Magnetic resonance (MR) contrast agents, 189-207
    dosage of, for neonates and infants, 198-199
    double-dose regimens of, 204-205
    ferrites as, 206-207
    gadolinium-based; *see* Gadolinium (Gd) based contrast agents
    gastrointestinal, 205-206
    half-dose regimens of, 204-205
    hepatic, 207
    high-dose regimens of, 204-205
    newer, safety of, 203
    particulate agents as, 206-207
    pregnant or lactating women and, 205
    relaxation rates after administration of, 189, 190
    selection of patients for, 203-204
    superparamagnetic iron oxide crystals as, 206-207
    triple-dose regimens of, 204-205
    water-soluble, 206
Magnetic resonance imaging (MRI), 23, 79-111
    advanced techniques of, 208-239
    brightness of vessel in, 165-166
    contraindications to, 240-260
    conventional spin echo imaging and, 237-238
    dangers of, 240
    diffusion imaging and, 231-232
    echo planar imaging and, 238-239
    effect of, on EKG, 255-256
    fast spin echo imaging and, 233-238
    "fat sat" pulses in, 212-214
    fat suppression in, 210-212, 216-217
    fractional echo imaging and, 226-227
    fractional NEX imaging and, 226-227
    hydrogen spectroscopy and, 218-220
    magnetic field strengths used for, 62-63
    versus magnetic resonance spectroscopy, 217-218

Magnetic resonance imaging (MRI)—cont'd
  magnetization transfer imaging technique of, 208-210
  partial Fourier imaging and, 224-225, 226
  phase conjugate symmetry technique and, 227-228
  phase-offset multiplanar imaging and, 223-224
  phosphorous spectroscopy and, 220-223
  read conjugate symmetry technique and, 227-228
  rectangular field of view and, 228-231
  safety and biological effects of, 240-260
  sedation of infants and children for, 251-252
  short T1 inversion recovery in, 214-216
  urban legends of, 240
  variable bandwidth technique and, 232, 233
Magnetic resonance (MR) scanners
  classification of, 62-63
  4.0 T, biological effects and, 257-258
  hardware, 62-78
  high- and low-field, 62-63
  horizontal-field; *see* Horizontal-field magnets
  loudness of, 253-254
  north and south poles of, 4
  1.5-tesla, 3
  permanent, 64
  resistive, 65
  specifications for gradients and, 67
  strength of, 1-3
  superconducting, 64
  tasks carried out by, during prescan period, 75-76
  turning off, 64-65
  vertical-field, 3, 4, 63
Magnetic resonance (MR) signal channels, 71-72
Magnetic resonance spectroscopy (MRS), 3, 23, 217-218
Magnetic susceptibility, 7, 145, 146, 147
Magnetic susceptibility gradient, 14
Magnetically activated implants, 242
Magnetically activated tissue expanders, 250
Magnetism and electricity, basic principles of, 1-21
Magnetizability, 9
Magnetization, 7-8, 9, 32-33
Magnetization transfer (MT) imaging, 208-210, 237
Magnetization transfer ratio (MTR), 209-210
Magnetization-prepared GRE techniques, 118, 132-133
Magnetizing force, 6
Magnetohydrodynamics, effect of MR scanner on EKG and, 256
Magnetophosphenes, 4.0 T MR scanner and, 258
Magnevist; *see* Gd-DTPA/dimeglumine
Magnitude image, 71-72, 73-74
Makeup, eye, MR imaging and, 246
Manganese dipyridoxal diphosphate, 207
Mannitol as bowel MR contrast agent, 206
Mascara, MR imaging and, 246

Mass susceptibilities, 8
Matter, magnetic properties of, 10, 11
Maximum gradient strength, MR scanners and, 67
Maximum intensity projection (MIP) reconstruction, TOF MR angiography and, 181
McGee platinum stainless steel piston, 247
Measurements, signal-to-noise ratio and, 107
Metal fragments, intraocular, movement of, during MR scan, 245-246
Metal heart valves, MR imaging and, 244-245
Metallic implants, 241-242
Metallic shrapnel, MR imaging and, 248-249
Meter-kilogram-second-ampere (MKSA) system, 1
Microwave ovens, safety of, 258-259
Middle ear prostheses, MR imaging and, 247
Midfield MR scanners, 62, 63
Military shrapnel, MR imaging and, 248-249
Misregistration, eddy currents and, 68
Molar susceptibilities, 8
Molecular diffusion, 231-232
Molecular tumbling rate, relationship between T1 or T2 and, 37, 38
Monitoring devices, MR-compatible, 252-253
Motion artifact suppression technique (MAST), 176-178
Motion artifacts, 155-157
MP-RAGE, 133
Multiple overlapping thin-slab acquisition (MOTSA), 185-186
Myelin-related amino acids, hydrogen spectroscopy and, 220

N

N-acetylaspartate (NAA), hydrogen spectroscopy and, 218, 220
β-NAG, elevation of, Gd-DTPA and, 199
Nembutal; *see* Pentobarbital
Net nuclear magnetization, spins represented as, 33
Neurosurgical devices, MR imaging and, 242
Nitrogen
  gaseous, escape of, during quench, 66
  liquid, in superconducting MR scanners, 65
Noise, image, white, 107, 108
Nonferromagnetic bullets, 248-249
Nonionic gadolinium-based contrast agents; *see* Gadolinium-based contrast agents, nonionic
Nonionic iodine contrast agents, 203
No-phase-wrap software, phase wraparound artifacts and, 151
No-phase-wrap technique, 151-152, 153, 223
North pole of MR scanner, 4
Nuclear induction, 23, 33
Nuclear magnetic resonance (NMR), 12, 22-61
  Bloch equations and, 33-36
  chemical shifts and, 49-52
  classical model of, 22-23
  dipole-dipole interactions and, 44-47
  free induction decay and, 52-56
  nuclei and, 24-26

Nuclear magnetic resonance (NMR)—cont'd
    protons and, 24-29
    quantum mechanical model of, 22-23
    spin echo and, 53-56
    spins and, 24-26, 29-30
    stimulated echo and, 59-60
    T1 relaxation and, 37, 38
    T2 relaxation and, 38-39
Nuclear paramagnetic resonance, 23
Nuclear paramagnetism, 12
Nuclear spin, 24-26
Nuclei, nuclear magnetic resonance and, 24-26
Null point, STIR sequence and, 214, 215
Number of excitations (NEX), 107
Nurse, presence of, in scanner room, 253
Nyquist frequency, 152

O

Ocular implants, MR imaging and, 242
Ocular prostheses, 242, 246
Odd echo dephasing, 166, 174, 175
Oersted (Oe), 7
Omniscan; *see* Gadodiamide
Orbital foreign body, movement of, 245-246
Orthopedic appliances, MR imaging and, 242
Otologic implants, MR imaging and, 242
Oversampling, signal, 154
Oximeter, pulse, for monitoring patient, 252-253

P

Pacemakers, MR imaging and, 242, 243-244
Palatal nerve stimulation, 4.0 T MR scanner
    and, 258
Palpebral springs, eyelid, MR imaging and, 246
Papooselike restraints in reduction of ghost
    artifacts, 157-158
Paradoxical enhancement, slowly flowing blood
    and, 166, 167
Paramagnetic substances, 7-8, 10, 14
    specific relaxivities of, 190
Paramagnetism, 9, 11-14
Parallel and antiparallel states, quantum me-
    chanics and, 25
Partial flip angle pulse, 114-115
Partial flip angles, 114-115, 116-117
Partial Fourier imaging, 224-225, 226
Particulate agents as liver MR contrast agents,
    206-207
Passive shimming, 67
Patient
    anesthetized, monitoring of, 252-253
    claustrophobic, interventions for, 250-251
    critically ill, monitoring of, 252-253
    pregnant; *see* Pregnant patient
    selection of, for administration of MR con-
        trast agents, 203-204
Peak gradient strength, MR scanners and, 67
Pellets, MR imaging and, 248-249
Penile prostheses, MR imaging and, 250
Pentobarbital (Nembutal) in sedation of infants
    and children, 251

Permanent MR magnet, 64
Permeability of free space, 6-7, 9
Phase, 19-22
Phase angle, steady state free precession and, 123
Phase artifacts, 172-173
Phase conjugate symmetry, 224-225, 227-228, 229
Phase contrast (PC) MR angiography versus
    time-of-flight MR angiography, 181-183
Phase encoding, 87, 88, 90-92, 97, 178-181
Phase evolution of fat suppression, 210-212
Phase image, MR signal channels and, 72, 73-74
Phase shifts, 93-94
Phase wraparound, 145-151
Phase wraparound artifacts, software for elimi-
    nating, 151
Phased-array coil, 72-75
Phased-array systems, true, 75
Phase-encode direction
    chemical shift artifacts and, 138-139
    motion artifacts and, 155
Phase-encoding gradient, 91, 92
Phase-offset multiplanar (POMP) imaging, 152,
    223-224
Phase-reordering methods in reduction of ghost
    artifacts, 157-158
Phenergan; *see* Demerol, Thorazine, and Phen-
    ergan cocktail
Phosphocreatine (PCr)
    hydrogen spectroscopy and, 220
    phosphorous spectroscopy and, 221-222
Phosphodiesters (PDE), phosphorous spectros-
    copy and, 221
Phosphomonoesters (PME), phosphorous spec-
    troscopy and, 221
Phosphorescence, spontaneous emission of en-
    ergy and, 29
Phosphorous spectroscopy, 220-223
Physical restraint of body motion in reduction
    of ghost artifacts, 157-158
Pixel, 93-94, 97
    size of, 91, 101-106
    values of, 94-98
Planck's law, quantum mechanics and, 25
Plug flow, 164
Poppen-Blaylock carotid artery vascular clamp,
    MR imaging and, 250
Power lines, safety of, 259-260
Precession, gyroscopic, 16-19
Precession angle, 123
Precessional frequency, 19
Precompensation, eddy currents and, 68, 69
Precordial stethoscope for monitoring patient
    during MR scan, 252-253
Preemphasis, eddy currents and, 68, 69
Pregnant patient
    gadolinium-based contrast agents given to, 205
    MR imaging of, 254-255
Pregnant technologist, risk to, 255
Preparatory pulses, 133
Prescan, tasks carried out by MR scanner dur-
    ing, 75-76

ProHance; *see* Gadoteridol
Proton-electron dipole-dipole interactions, 44
Proton-proton dipole-dipole interaction, 44
Protons
    action of, within magnetic field, 16-18
    aliphatic, chemical shifts of, 50
    deshielded, 49
    expectation value of, 28
    hydrogen, in water molecule, nuclear para-
        magnetism of, 12
    in lower energy state, 29
    nuclear magnetic resonance and, 24-26
    shielded, 49
    spinor property of, 32-33
    in spin-up and spin-down states, 25, 26-28, 29
    wave-particle duality of, 27
Prudent avoidance, electromagnetic fields and,
    258-259
Pseudolayering, 192, 193
PSIF versus FISP, 131-132
Pulse amplitude calibration in prescan, 77
Pulse flipping, 57, 58-59
Pulse oximeter for monitoring patient, 252-253

Q

Quadrature coil design, 70-71
Quadrature detection, 70-71
Quadrature signal detection, 98
Quadrupolar moment, 48
Quadrupolar relaxation, 48
Quadrupole-electrical field interaction, T1 and
    T2 and, 48
Quantum mechanics, nuclear magnetic reso-
    nance and, 24-28
Quench, superconducting scanners and, 64-66

R

Radiation, electromagnetic, prolonged exposure
    to, effect of, on fetus, 254-255
Ramping up and ramping down superconduct-
    ing scanners, 64-65
Rapid acquisition with refocused echoes
    (RARE) technique, 233-235
Rapid SE imaging, 233-235
Read conjugate symmetry, phase conjugate
    symmetry and, 227-228, 229
Read symmetry, 226-227
Readout gradient, 88
Readout lobe, 88
Real MR signal channels, 71-72, 73-74
Real-time acquisition and velocity evaluation
    (RACE), 186
Receive attenuator adjustment, 77-78
Receiver bandwidth (BW), 88-89, 107-108
Rectangular field of view (FOV), 101, 228-231
Relative magnetic permeability, 7, 9
Relaxation
    quadrupolar, 48
    spin-spin, 38
    T1, 35, 36, 37, 38, 39, 41
    T2, 35, 36, 38-39, 40

Relaxation properties of tissues, 42-44
Relaxation rates after contrast administration,
    189, 190
Relaxation time, 37, 38-39
Remanence, ferromagnetism and, 13
Renal failure or insufficiency, gadolinium-based
    contrast agents and, 199-200
Renograffin-60, total osmolar load from, 203
Rephasing
    even echo, 166, 174-176
    gradient motion, 176-178
Resistive MR scanners, 65
Resonance phenomenon, 32
Resonant offset angle, steady state free preces-
    sion and, 123, 124, 125-126
Resonant offset averaging, elimination of
    FLASH bands and, 125-126
Resonex RX 5000HP, 65
Respirators, 252-253
Respiratory comp in reduction of ghost arti-
    facts, 157-158
Respiratory gating in reduction of ghost arti-
    facts, 157-158
Resuscitation equipment, administration of gad-
    olinium and, 195-196
Retinal tack, MR imaging and, 246
Rewinder gradients, elimination of FLASH
    bands and, 125-126
Reynold's number, turbulence and, 164
RF flip angle, 30
RF pulse, 58
RF spoiling, 119
RF transmitter bandwidth, 89, 107
RF-FAST, 119
Ringing artifacts, 142-144
Rise time, gradient strength and, MR scanners
    and, 67
ROPE in reduction of ghost artifacts, 157-158

S

Saddle coils, horizontal-field magnets and, 63
Safety of MR imaging, 240-260
Saturation, 167
Scalar coupling, T1 and T2 and, 47
Scanners; *see* Magnetic resonance (MR) scanners
Schrödinger equation, 27
Secular contribution to T2, 39
Sedation of infants and children, 251-252
Sequential multislice acquisition, 130-131
Shavers, electric, safety of, 258-259
Shielded gradients, eddy currents and, 68
Shielded protons, 49
Shielding, gradient, 69
Shimming, 67
Short T1 inversion recovery (STIR)
    elimination of chemical shift artifacts in rou-
        tine spin warp imaging and, 140
    fat suppression and, 210, 214-216
Shotgun pellets, MR imaging and, 248-249
Shrapnel, 242, 248-249
SI; *see* Système International d'Unites

Signa, 64
Signal channels, MR, 71-72
Signal intensity of spin echo imaging as
    function of gadolinium concentration,
    192
Signal oversampling, 154
Signal-to-noise ratio (SNR)
    calculation of, 106-109
    cross-talk and, 86
    improvement of, by adjusting imaging pa-
        rameters, 109
    of magnetic resonance spectroscopy, 218
    for 3DFT, 108, 109-110
    for 2DFT, 108, 109-110
    VENC and, 183
Sinc function, Fourier transform and, 81, 82
Sine wave, 19-22, 79-80, 81
Skin perfusion monitor for patient, 252-253
Skin staples, MR imaging and, 243
Slice-interleaved acquisition, 131
Slice-multiplexed acquisition, 130-131
Slice-selective excitation, 82-84
Slice-selective gradient reversal, 210, 216-217
Software for eliminating phase wraparound
    artifacts, 151
Solenoidal coils, vertical-field magnets and,
    63
South pole of MR scanner, 4
Spatial blurring, eddy currents and, 68
Specific absorption rate (SAR), 71, 256
Spectral leakage artifacts, 142-144
Spectroscopic techniques of fat suppression,
    216-217
Spectroscopy
    clinical, localization methods in, 218, 219
    depth-related surface coil, 219
    hydrogen, 218-220
    image selected in vivo, 219
    magnetic resonance, 23, 217-218
    phosphorous, 220-223
    water-suppressed hydrogen, 52
SPGR, 119, 133
Spin echo (SE), 61
    versus free induction decay, 53-56
    versus gradient echo, 112-113
    steady state free precession and, 122-125
Spin echo (SE) imaging
    chemical shift artifacts and, 140-141
    versus fast spin echo imaging, 237-238
    signal intensity of, as function of gadolinium
        concentration, 192
    T2-shortening effects of gadolinium during,
        191-193
Spin isochromat, 25-26, 55
Spin quantum number, 24-26
Spin warp imaging, chemical shift artifacts and,
    139-140
Spin-lattice interactions, 53
Spin-lattice relaxation time, 37
Spinor property of protons, 32-33
Spin-phase effects, 170-171

Spins
    in higher-energy levels, 29-30
    nuclear magnetic resonance and, 24-26
Spin-spin interactions, 53
Spin-spin relaxation, 38
Spin-up and spin-down states, quantum me-
        chanics and, 25, 26-28, 29
Spoiled GRE, 118, 119-121, 126, 128
    versus conventional short TR/TE spin echo
        sequences, 121-122
    manipulating image contrast in, 120
Spoiling, 118-119
Spontaneous emission of energy, 29-30
Springs, eyelid palpebral, 246
SSFP, 131-132
SS-GRE-FID sequences, 126
SS-GRE-SE sequences, 126
Starr-Edwards valves, pre-6000 series, 244-245
Static field inhomogeneities, 5, 53
Steady-state coherent sequences, 126-127
Steady-state free precession, 122-125, 126-127,
        131-132
Steady-state GRE, 118
Steady-state incoherent sequences, 126-127
Stethoscope, precordial, for monitoring patient
        during MR scan, 252-253
Stimulated echo (STE), 59-60, 61
    steady state free precession and, 122-125
Stimulated echo acquisition mode (STEAM), 60,
        219
Superconducting MR scanners, 64
Super-high-field MR scanners, 62
Superparamagnetic iron oxide crystals as liver
        MR contrast agents, 206-207
Superparamagnetism, 10, 11
    versus paramagnetism and ferromagnetism,
        12-14
Suppression
    fat; *see* Fat suppression
    of signal from tissue generating ghost arti-
        facts, 157-158
Surgical clips, MR imaging and, 243
Surgiclips, 243
Susceptibility artifacts, 145, 146, 147
Susceptibility distortions, 145, 146, 147
Susceptibility gradients, 5
    magnetic, 14
Swan-Ganz catheters, MR imaging and, 242
Swan-Ganz thermodilution catheters, 249-250
Switchable arrays, 75
SynchroMed pump, MR imaging and, 244
Système International d'Unites (SI), 1
Systolic blood flow velocities, peak, 163

T

T1
    of different tissues, prediction of, 42-44
    as function of field strength, 40-41
T2
    of different tissues, prediction of, 42-44
    secular contribution to, 39

T2—cont'd
  versus T2*, 41-42
  value of, as function of field strength, 40-41
T2*; *see* T2-star
T2 decay processes, 56
T2* decay processes, 53
T1 relaxation, 35, 36, 37, 38, 39, 41
T2 relaxation, 35, 36, 38-39, 40
T1 weighting, 110-111, 129, 130
T2 weighting, 110-111, 129, 130
Tattoos, eyelid, MR imaging and, 246
Technologist
  pregnant, risk to, 255
  to monitor patient during MR scan, 253
"Tech-retary," 255
Temperature monitor for patient, 252-253
Temperature stability, magnet field homogene-
    ities and, 66
Tesla (T), 1-3
Tetraazacyclododecane tetraacetic acid (DOTA),
    201
Tetramethylsilane (TMS)
  chemical shifts and, 49-50
  hydrogen spectroscopy and, 218
T1-FAST, 119
Thermal relaxation time, 37
Thorazine; *see* Demerol, Thorazine, and Phener-
    gan cocktail
Thorotrast, 207
3D-FATS; *see* Water-selective excitation
3DFT, signal-to-noise ratio and, 108, 109-110
3/4-NEX imaging, 225
THRIFT, 117
Thrombus, distinguishing slow flow from, 172-
    174
Time-of-flight (TOF) effects, 166-169
Time-of-flight (TOF) MR angiography
  magnetization transfer imaging and, 209
  versus phase contrast MR angiography, 181-
    183
Tissue expanders
  magnetically activated, MR imaging and, 250
  MR imaging and, 242
TMS; *see* Tetramethylsilane
Topping off of cryogens in superconducting MR
    scanners, 65
Torque experienced by spins, 33
Transcutaneous electrical stimulation (TENS),
    244
Transfusion pumps, implanted, 244
Transmit attenuation adjustment in prescan, 77
Transmitter leakage, zipperlike artifacts and,
    159-160
Transverse relaxation time, 38-39
Triangular waveform, decomposition of, into
    principal components, 79-80

Truncation artifacts, 142-144
Truncation errors, 80, 142-144
T1-shortening effects of gadolinium, 191-193
T2-shortening effects of gadolinium, 191-193
T2-star (T2*) versus T2, 41-42
Turbo-FLASH versus FLASH, 132-133
Turbo-SE imaging, 233-235
Turbulence, Reynold's number and, 164
Turbulent flow, 163-165
2DFT, signal-to-noise ratio and, 108, 109-110

U

Ultra-high-field MR scanners, 62
Ultra-low-field MR scanners, 62
Urban legends of MR imaging, 240

V

Variable bandwidth technique, 232, 233
Velocity aliasing, VENC and, 184
Velocity encoding (VENC), phase contrast MR
    angiography and, 182, 183-185
Velocity imaging in a cine mode (VINNIE), 187
Vertical-field magnets, 3, 4, 63
Very-low-field MR scanners, 62
Volume magnetic susceptibility, 7, 9
Vortex flow, 163-165
Voxel, 101-106

W

Washing machines, safety of, 258-259
Water
  bound, 37, 42
  bulk content of, T1 and T2 values and, 42-43
  chemical shift of, 50
  diamagnetism of, 12
  and fat protons, chemical shift between, 138-
    139
  free, 37, 42
  molecule of, hydrogen protons in, nuclear
    paramagnetism of, 12
  structured, 37, 42
Water-selective excitation (3D-FATS), fat sup-
    pression and, 210, 216-217
Water-soluble MR contrast agents, 206
Water-suppressed hydrogen spectroscopy, 52
Wave function, protons and, 27, 28
White image noise, 107, 108
Wires, MR imaging and, 242
Wraparound artifacts, 152-154
Wraparound coils, 63

Z

Zeeman energy levels, 24-25, 26-28
Zipperlike artifacts, 159-160